D0621477

The
Joys of
Pediatrics

Editor
Mohsen Ziai, MD, Honorary FAAP

Foreword by
Robert J. Haggerty, MD, FAAP

American Academy of Pediatrics
141 Northwest Point Blvd
Elk Grove Village, IL 60007

AAP Publishing Staff

Director, Department of Marketing and Publications
Maureen DeRosa, MPA

Director, Division of Product Development
Mark Grimes

Manager, Product Development
Jeff Mahony

Director, Division of Publishing and Production Services
Sandi King

Manager, Editorial Services
Kate Larson

Manager, Print Production Services
Leesa Levin-Doroba

Manager, Graphic Design
Linda Diamond

Director, Division of Marketing and Sales
Jill Ferguson

Manager, Publication and Program Marketing
Linda Smessaert

Library of Congress Control Number: 2004102272
ISBN: 1-58110-141-4
MA0284

Patient names used within this publication have been changed, and certain story elements have been modified for readability. The information contained in this publication is for the reader's enjoyment only and should not be used as a substitute for the medical care and advice of your pediatrician. There may be variations in treatment that your pediatrician may recommend based on individual facts and circumstances. Some medical practices described in this publication may no longer be or may never have been recommended methods of treatment. Though care has been taken to ensure the originality of all submissions, the American Academy of Pediatrics is not responsible for the inclusion of anecdotes that may also appear elsewhere in similar forms.

Reviewers/Contributors

Editor
Mohsen Ziai, MD, Honorary FAAP

Assistant Editor
Parinaz Ziai Bahadori

Foreword
Robert J. Haggerty, MD, FAAP

AAP Board of Directors Reviewer
Charles W. Linder, MD, FAAP

American Academy of Pediatrics
Executive Director/CEO
Errol R. Alden, MD, FAAP

Immediate Past Executive Director
Joe M. Sanders, Jr, MD, FAAP

Associate Executive Director
Roger F. Suchyta, MD, FAAP

Director, Department of Marketing and Publications
Maureen DeRosa, MPA

Director, Division of Product Development
Mark Grimes

Manager, Product Development
Jeff Mahony

Manager, Editorial Services
Kate Larson

Dedicated to children everywhere, and the people who care for them.

Table of Contents

Preface

As health care professionals, we are blessed through daily personal human interactions. Children are particularly important in this respect because they constitute our only link with the future of mankind. Additionally, their courage, sense of humor, and appreciation of love more than make up for our devotion to their welfare—these rewards exceed any possible financial compensation.

As a pediatrician, teacher, and health care provider for half a century, I have many memories from my professional life dedicated to the well-being of children and their families. Almost 3 years ago I was recounting some of these stories, as well as other anecdotes, that I had heard over the years to my daughter, Parinaz. She enjoyed these very much and suggested contacting other colleagues to collect their memories for the publication of a book.

I discussed these ideas with my distinguished friend and colleague, Robert J. Haggerty, MD. He approved of the idea, and because of his intimate relationship with the American Academy of Pediatrics (AAP) as a past president, he made arrangements for the publication of what we had already gathered. Their decision fulfilled our wishes to use this book as a vehicle to promote an understanding of the unique pleasure of taking care of children by an organization that has been successfully involved on behalf of children for 75 years.

We hope this book will motivate other contributions from many more caretakers of children for future publications.

Parinaz's efforts have constituted the backbone of our success, but the generous input of numerous contributors has resulted in the realization of our dream. The support of Dr Haggerty and numerous individuals at the AAP, including Jeff Mahony, Mark Grimes, and Maureen DeRosa, deserve our highest gratitude. We know that they will be rewarded by the appreciation of those who have a chance to read these memorable stories.

Mohsen Ziai, MD, Honorary FAAP
Editor

Foreword

"Out of the mouths of babes" is a common saying to indicate that children, unfettered by adult convention, speak the unvarnished truth. They are often funny, when they take events or the words of adults literally; sometimes sad, when a child with a fatal disease receives bad news without flinching; and always courageous, when a child faces death with equanimity. Such are the sayings of children that Dr Mohsen Ziai and his daughter, Parinaz, have assembled from many pediatricians. Humor makes the difficult days go better. Reading these anecdotes will give everyone a chuckle that will make their days a bit lighter. Some of the courageous sayings of very ill children will bring tears to the eyes of every reader and help them and parents face difficult times with more serenity.

Any experienced physician will remember similar sayings of their patients. Dr Ziai hopes that they will send him more such "out of the mouths of babes" tales so that other editions of these sayings can be recorded for future physicians and parents, for both are the audience for such a book. Dr Ziai has an especially sensitive ear for children's feelings. Reading these anecdotes will help other physicians develop their sensitive ear. I believe every resident physician will benefit from reading these anecdotes, gaining a bit of the wisdom of children and learning to listen a bit more perceptively to them. Physicians are often criticized for talking too much to their patients. Reading this book will help us all listen more and talk less.

I urge all physicians who deal with children to read this book, share these sayings with others, and enjoy the wisdom that comes "out of the mouths of babes."

Robert J. Haggerty, MD, FAAP
Professor and Chair, Emeritus
University of Rochester School of Medicine
and Dentistry
Past President, American Academy of Pediatrics

Chapter 1

Kids Say the Darndest Things

Part I

When examining a young boy for his 5-year-old check-up, I was listening to his heart with my stethoscope. After diligently listening at each of the prescribed locations, my young patient asked, "What's the matter Doctor, can't you find it?"

Diane Dubinsky, MD
Fairfax, VA

℘

As a general pediatrics fellow in Michigan, I see kids in a pediatric clinic in a domestic violence shelter. Many of the children who are temporarily housed in the shelter have some nutritional issues that we try to address in the clinic.

I was doing a well-child exam on a 4-year-old boy in the clinic, and he was playing on the floor with some toys. I asked his mom, "How does he eat?" (Meaning, what sort of dietary patterns does he have and what is the nutritional content of his food.)

The little boy, taking my question quite literally, turned to me and proudly said, "I eat with my hands!"

That comment just made my day!

Sandy Jee, MD
Ann Arbor, MI

A 5-year-old patient came into the examining room carrying a wooden toy hammer. When I finally persuaded him to climb up on the examining table, he gave the hammer to his dad and said, "Hit him, Dad."

James E. Strain, MD
Denver, CO

∅

I have a precocious 4-year-old patient who came into the office to tell me a joke. My previous experience with jokes told by patients this age is that either they aren't funny or the patient can't remember them. I was surprised to find myself laughing out loud at this young boy's joke. Every time I tell it, the children and the adults laugh.

Michael: "What is a caterpillar afraid of?"

Dr Baucom: "I don't know, what is a caterpillar afraid of?"

Michael: "A dogerpiller!"

Sandra Baucom, MD
Chesapeake, VA

∅

One night I was seeing an outgoing 8-year-old girl with upper respiratory infection symptoms. While doing my review of systems I asked her if her tummy hurt her, and she said very quickly and seriously, "Only when I jump up real high and land on my tummy on something sharp on the ground."

Well, that's not exactly what I'd meant, but it was a true answer and it made me laugh.

Christine White, MD
Kansas City, MO

℘

The smiling 4-year-old boy was very talkative as I entered the exam room. I identified myself and asked what had brought him to the doctor. Before his father could answer, the 4-year-old said, "I have a worm in my stomach."

His father was not born in the United States, so I was not completely confident about dismissing his medical history. When I gave the father a quizzical look, he raised his shoulders and smiled. I relaxed and began to examine the child's abdomen. "It's on the inside, not the outside," he stated.

"Why do you have a worm in your stomach?" I asked.

"Because I eat too much candy," he replied.

I countered with, "I guess you'll have to stop eating all that candy."

He looked at me very seriously and said, "I can't."

When I asked why, he smiled and said, "I need to feed the worm."

Unknown contributor

Asking a teenaged girl to lose weight, I suggested that she cut down on soda and candy and that she have a sandwich at noon and in the evening with a salad.

She said, "Doctor, cutting down on soda and candy is no problem, but the sandwiches…should I take them before or after meals?"

John G. Bitar, MD
McLean, VA

⌇

I was working in Stuttgart, Germany, as the head nurse in the pediatric clinic. In the mornings the pediatrician and I ran a sick call. One morning my neighbor brought in her 3-year-old son because of a sore throat. While I was getting David's vital signs, his mom started laughing and telling me what David had said as she was getting him ready to come to the clinic. David had put on his shoes, and when he came into the room to see his mother, she had looked down and said, "David, you have your shoes on the wrong feet." He looked at his feet and then looked at his mom and said, "They're the only feet I have."

Mary Williamson, RN
Falls Church, VA

⌇

For Take Your Daughter to Work Day I took my 12-year-old daughter with me to the neonatal intensive care unit for the morning. Among the patients was a baby that required an exchange transfusion. After I put my daughter on the bus home, I called my wife. My wife assured me that our daughter had arrived home safely, but that she was very concerned because she had overheard me explaining to a mother that her baby required a "sex change."

Ronald Pye, MD
Boston, MA

℘

A mother brought in her 4-year-old because she was concerned about his hearing. Using an audiometer, I determined that the child's hearing acuity was excellent at all frequencies. After I related the finding to the mother, the little boy said very seriously, "I always hear her, but sometimes I just don't want to answer."

Carl A. Salsbury, MD
Falls Church, VA

℘

On one occasion I was scheduled to attend a college graduation ceremony where I was to receive an honorary degree. When the subject was mentioned in the presence of my little granddaughter she remarked, "Granddaddy is already a Phi Baby Kappa!"

Edwin Lawrence Kendig, Jr, MD
Richmond, VA

I am a pediatrician in a small town, lucky to be blessed with 3 sons and a wonderful husband who can fix anything. My middle son, David, was about 4 and was at a friend's house that he frequented regularly. The mom of the house, Fefe, was fixing a screen door and the two 4-year-olds were "helping."

David to Fefe: "You can't fix that."

Fefe: "Why not?"

David: "Only dads fix doors."

Fefe: "Well, what do moms do?"

David: "They are doctors!"

Joan E. Flender, MD
Dansville, NY

℘

With my name being "Schweisthal," it has been pronounced many ways. One of the ways I have enjoyed the most was when a 4-year-old boy called me "Dr Sweat Socks."

Paul Schweisthal, MD
Vienna, VA

℘

At the onset of signs of puberty in our patients, my colleagues and I ordinarily scheduled extra time with each patient and provided some basic sexuality education. Our streetwise patients often would deny any knowledge, presumably to see if what I told them matched what they had heard before. One young lady truly did have some confusion about the "birds and the bees." After we were done discussing ovulation, fertilization, etc, she was asked if she had any questions.

She nodded, "Only one. What happens to the eggshell?"

Edward L. Schor, MD
Des Moines, IA

✆

While listening to a 4-year-old's heart during a routine physical, I thought I'd get him engaged in the process. I asked him, "Do you know what your heart says?" After a brief pause, he answered, "My heart says, 'Jesus loves me!'" A spontaneous statement of faith.

Majdi M. Abu-Salih, MD
Hartford, WI

✆

In the middle of an office visit, a mother took one of her children to the bathroom, leaving me with the 5-year-old sister.

"So," I said to the sister, "are you in kindergarten?"

"Yes," she said proudly, "and I really like it."

"What do you do there?" I asked.

"We do projects. Right now we are studying the rain forest."

I replied, "Tell me about the rain forest."

"Well," she said, "there are lots of plants there, and lots of animals."

"Where is the rain forest?" I asked. "Is it nearby?"

"Oh no," she laughed. "It's very, very far away… maybe in Buffalo!"

The next time you see a parrot flying over the New York Thruway, it probably came from the Buffalo rain forest.

Lawrence F. Nazarian, MD
Rochester, NY

☙

Years ago we routinely did tuberculosis tests for kindergarten entrance physicals. Late one morning I finished examining an adorable 5-year-old and proceeded to tell him about what he and my nurses would be doing next. "When I leave here, Penny will come in. She'll play a game with you where you tell her what pictures you see, and you'll listen to beeps in some headphones so we can check your hearing. Then she'll help you stay healthy by giving you something in a little bottle to drink, a shot in each arm, and a tuberculosis test." The young man smiled, turned calmly to his mother and said, "Oh good. We haven't gone to Burger King yet; I'll pass the *toomanyburgerstest.*"

Joan E. Flender, MD
Dansville, NY

✆

Recently a 3-year-old patient who always brought his stuffed octopus with him forgot and left it in the car. I was teasing him about the octopus driving his van around the parking lot. He jumped up from the table and ran to look out the window. At that moment, there was a van exactly like his driving around. The patient looked up at me and said, "It only takes two hands to drive. I don't know what he is doing with the other six, but he better not be eating my Halloween candy."

Stephen P. Combs, MD
Gray, TN

Chapter 2

Parent Parade
Part I

With my parents of challenging toddlers, I like to frame the behavior in a positive light, telling them that usually the smartest kids are the ones that give the parents the most trouble. As the dad grabbed his son as he tried to escape from the exam table he commented, "If that's the case, this kid's going to be Einstein!"

Gail S. Hertz, MD
York, PA

❡

A father called our office in a panic. He reported to us that his son had a 104-degree temperature. We asked him how he took the temperature, and the father replied that he was quite shaken by such a fever but was getting himself under control!

Jim Baugh, MD
Fairfax, VA

❡

A young child had been up crying through the night. Suspecting an ear infection, I had to restrain this unhappy tot on my exam table to examine his ears. As I leaned over I observed drainage coming from his ear. So I took a curette and as I began pulling out some moist, cheesy, purulent material from the ear I mumbled something like, "(It) drained." Moments later I looked up and noted the mom to appear very anxious. "Did you say '*brain?*'" she asked.

Doug McDowall, MD
Fairfax, VA

A 12-week-old infant was brought to the emergency department by his maternal grandfather for concerns of nasal congestion. The grandfather was quite attentive to the baby and explained he was filling in as the baby's caregiver while the mother was away at a job-training meeting.

The elderly gentleman had become concerned when, earlier that day, the baby began making loud breathing noises. As I progressed in taking the history and observing the baby in his grandfather's arms, it became clear that the baby was not acutely ill. Overall, the grandfather was a good historian and could easily relate, in a simplistic but clear manner, the baby's status over the past couple of days. When I inquired regarding the birth history he became a little flustered.

"Where was the baby born?"

"Here, at this hospital."

"How much did the baby weigh?"

"A little over eight pounds."

"Any problems during his mother's pregnancy?"

"Don't think so."

"Was he born vaginally or by cesarean section?"

Pause… "You know, the regular way."

I could tell he was getting a little uncomfortable with this part of the history.

"Was he born close to his due date?"

"A little late."

Another pause…"And his mother had to be *seduced*."

"Seduced?" I asked.

"Yup, they had to give her some medicine to start her contractions."

"How long was the baby in the hospital?"

"Two days."

Long and short of the story…the baby was healthy, and after a lengthy session of counseling and anticipatory guidance, the grandfather left with peace of mind, with respect to the baby's medical condition and his mother's delivery history.

Robert J. Swantz, MD
Rochester, NY

✇

Mrs Baker had 6 children and was a patient of mine for many years. I started to see her and her children in the early days of my practice when I was not busy and, even though she lived 20 miles from my office, I could easily make house calls to see her sick children.

One day she called and said that one of the children had a fever of 105 degrees. I suggested she come to the office. She readily agreed and when she got there, I examined the child and could find nothing wrong. I examined the child a second time and could still find nothing wrong. I looked in despair at Mrs Baker.

Finally, she looked at the child and at me and commented that she had brought the wrong child to the office. "No problem," I said, "just go home and come back with the right one."

Solomon J. Cohen, MD
New York, NY

One day during Christmas week I received a long-distance phone call from a father at Disney World concerned about his 3-year-old son's fever. I explained to the father that I could not possibly diagnose and treat his son over the phone, and I told him to seek medical care at the Magic Kingdom where there is a walk-in clinic. He in return asked me to call in an antibiotic. "After all," he explained, "what is a little amoxicillin between friends?"

Ira S. Rubin, MD
Naperville, IL

℧

A large part of my pediatric clientele is Vietnamese, and it is easier for them and for me to speak Vietnamese during our encounters. The formula name *Nursoy* sounds almost like *Nuoc soi*, which in Vietnamese means "boiling water."

I recommended *Nursoy* for this baby with formula intolerance. His young mother immigrated to the United States just recently and knew very little English. She seemed to be happy with my thorough assessment and nodded docilely to my recommendation.

On her way to the door, though, she wanted to ask me a last question: "Doctor, do I have to give him boiling water when it is still hot or do I have to wait until it cools down?"

Hien V. Ho, MD
Great Falls, VA

Our office needed to collect a urine sample from a young patient, so our nurse asked the mother to bring it in a plastic bag. Lo and behold, the mother placed her child in a plastic bag from the waist down to transport her into the office! We had a laugh about that one for a long time!

Ghassan Atiyeh, MD
Alexandria, VA

✄

I had an urgent telephone call from a mother who said her child had been bitten by an elephant. I couldn't quite understand this until she told me she was calling from a petting zoo.

James E. Strain, MD
Denver, CO

✄

There was a newborn baby brought to the outpatient department for a checkup, and I asked what the baby's name was. The reply was "Female."

I was puzzled and asked where that name came from, and she said, "I didn't think it up; it was on the birth certificate."

Mary Ellen Avery, MD
Boston, MA

In her first year of life a healthy girl was treated with amoxicillin for ear infections on 5 occasions when she presented to her physician with respiratory symptoms, sometimes with fever. Beginning with the third episode her physician suggested that ear tubes might be helpful for the recurrent otitis and residual middle-ear effusion. In the winter after she turned 12 months old, no additional diagnoses of acute otitis media were made and no more antibiotics were prescribed. At age 2½ years, in response to a query about what happened that resulted in the disappearance of otitis media, the mother's answer was, "I stopped taking her to the doctor for colds."

J. Owen Hendley, MD
Charlottesville, VA

I had repeatedly urged the mother of an infant with a high fever of unknown origin to be absolutely sure to call me no matter what time of day or night to let me know if the child was not doing well. At just about 3:00 am that night, sure enough, she called…to let me know that the baby was "much better." The mother was (I thought) so impressed with my genuine concern that she wanted to put my mind at ease. I feel certain that this is not a rare occurrence and that we must, indeed, make sure that parents of sick children have no hesitation about keeping in touch, even though some unnecessary calls will result.

Charles D. Cook, MD
Old Lyme, CT

When the hepatitis vaccine became available, my son, Eric, was most disappointed to hear that he had to undergo yet another series of immunizations. I explained to him the importance of the vaccine, and we somehow went off on a discussion of various forms of hepatitis and liver disease. As we were driving home after his last shot, he turned to me with a question. "Mom," he asked, "explain it to me again. Am I protected against seafood or sex?" I consider myself normally to be a very truthful person, but must admit that I replied to him that he was now free to eat an unlimited amount of seafood.

Dannie Huntington, MD
Falls Church, VA

A mother called in because her child had ingested some paint. She (the mother) was an artist and was doing a project. She suddenly became aware that her daughter had tasted the paint, and she needed advice fast. Before calling us, however, she too drank the paint to test it to see if it really was poisonous!

Jim Baugh, MD
Fairfax, VA

One Sunday afternoon I received a call from the father of one of my patients. He told me his son had severe abdominal pain. I told him that I was meeting someone else in the hospital and that he should meet me there. When I met him in the hospital, he informed me that he was not able to locate the son with the abdominal pain, so he decided to bring his other son instead!!

S. Mahallati, MD
Grasonville, MD

Chapter 3

Patient Breakthroughs
(Sometimes It's the Small Things)

I keep a supply of "negotiating tools" in my office, including candy dispensers (in various *Star Wars* characters), stickers, bubbles, popsicles, and pinwheels. A 5-year-old came in with florid strep throat. Her mom insisted she "get a shot" because the young girl would "never take the medicine." I saw this as a challenge. I sat with the "young lady" at the little plastic picnic table and together we colored in a *Little Mermaid* coloring book. We talked small talk for a while and I mentioned that when I had a sore throat I liked to drink things like tea. She suggested a tea party. In came the medicine cups (hers with amoxicillin and mine with juice), napkins, pinwheels, and stickers. Her mom called a few days later to say that their twice-a-day "tea party" is the highlight of their day.

Joan E. Flender, MD
Dansville, NY

℘

It was nearly 3:00 am when a mother called. I had barely lifted the phone from the cradle when an anxious voice shouted back, "Oh, I'm so glad you're home!"

She continued, "You treated my baby's rash last week and now it's gone."

Puzzled (and not a little bit irritated), I asked, "Why are you calling?"

"I can't sleep; I'm worried it might come back."

Angel Colon, MD
Bonita Springs, FL

When I was in pediatric practice in rural Upstate New York in the late 1950s, I was a member of a multispecialty group practice. When we were on call, we were expected to see all patients initially and call for help if we were unable to handle the situation. One wintry Saturday night I was on call for the group and received a call from a distraught man whose wife had started labor at home for their fourth child. He couldn't bring her to the hospital because we were having a blizzard, and the road they lived on was unplowed. I called the county sheriff's office and told them my predicament. They dispatched a highway department snowplow to my home, took me to the hospital where I picked up a home delivery kit, and proceeded to take me to the woman's home.

When we were about 2 miles from it, the plow ran into overwhelming drifts of snow and could not go farther. Fortunately, we were near a farmhouse and the farmer volunteered to take me cross-country on a wooden sleigh hooked up to a snowmobile that he used to haul hay during the winter months. I hopped on the sleigh and off we went, arriving without incident shortly thereafter. Covered from head to toe with snow, I knocked on the door. The now really harried husband greeted me with, "What took you so long, Doc?"

All went well, and a beautiful baby girl was born thanks to the sheriff, the highway department, and the friendly farmer.

Robert Hoekelman, MD
Rochester, NY

A colleague of mine (now deceased) was finishing a checkup visit for Amy, a 4-year-old preparing to enter preschool. As he wound up his assurances that Amy was normal, her mother said, "Oh by the way, Doctor, Bobby (Amy's 22-month-old little brother) doesn't seem to be able to hear."

The doctor asked how the mother came to know this, to which the mother replied that she assumed he couldn't hear because he never said anything. The doctor gathered additional information, such as whether Bobby could hear a candy wrapper being crinkled in the next room or the refrigerator door being opened 2 rooms away. The mother pointed out that Bobby was immediately alert following either of these auditory events. The doctor then inquired how Bobby was able to obtain what he wanted without speaking. The mother and Amy both suggested that he would take their hand and lead them to whatever he wanted, and his wishes were immediately gratified.

My colleague then spent 3 minutes reassuring the mother that it was clear that Bobby could hear, but that he may not be speaking because he had no need to with his older sister to look out for him. The look of disbelief in his mother's eyes stimulated my colleague to spend a further 2 minutes reiterating his message that Bobby was normal, but was not speaking because he did not need to. The mother remained unconvinced but agreed to wait and see for another month or two.

As the family left the exam room, Bobby turned back to the doctor, gave a wave of his hand and said, "Bye, Doc."

J. Owen Hendley, MD
Charlottesville, VA

An episode from the emergency department: A school-aged child and his mother came in to see me. He had his hand over his ear. His mother reported that if he took his hand away from his ear he had pain and heard a roaring sound. Indeed, when he removed his hand he complained of a great deal of pain. The otoscopic examination revealed the problem instantly. My bayonet forceps removed (yes, you guessed it!) a very large, very unhappy beetle trying to hide from the light. Mother and child were quite surprised and could not guess how this had occurred. But with the pain gone, the family left feeling happy and grateful. The hospital kept the bug.

David Bick, MD
Fairfax, VA

℘

I walked into the exam room to see Joe, a 17-year-old young man with a chief complaint of sore throat. We talked of college admissions, his interest in music, and non-interest in school. I turned to Joe and asked him how long he'd had a sore throat. He answered, and when I asked him to open his mouth he reluctantly said no. A little surprised, I informed him that without examining his throat I would not be able to give him any suggestions for treatment. Finally, he looked at me and said, "If I open my mouth, you won't tell my dad?" I promised and, lo and behold, a large tongue ring stared me in the face. I smiled and asked Joe how his father did not know about this. Joe looked baffled, as if I was truly ignorant and out of it. He never talked with his dad! After some discussion, Joe realized his dad probably knew about the ring and that it might be a way to let his dad get to know Joe a little better.

The next time I saw Joe, he said his dad was not surprised. Not only that, his dad had a new earring in place!

Mark J. Mendelsohn, MD
Charlottesville, VA

∅

A notoriously picky eater, I have given my family no end of troubles since childhood. Meals at home and out were always difficult because of the long list of items I was painfully afraid of trying. Now, as a pediatrician, I find myself relating more to my picky patients than to the beleaguered parents who complain about their child's diet. We often brainstorm together over creative ways to interest their child in trying new foods, but now and then I resort to my own methods.

The mother of 7-year-old Angelo was at her wits end, recalling for me every item on his "wild horses couldn't make me eat it" list of foods. She remarked that it was all the more surprising because his brothers were both such good eaters and always willing to try new things. Angelo watched me cautiously as I listened to his frustrated mother, wondering what drastic action I would recommend. I could tell this one wasn't going to be easy… Angelo clearly was taking this battle personally. I chuckled inside because I could relate so easily to his predicament. As his mom continued with her long list, I motioned to Angelo to come closer.

"So, Angelo, what do you have against mushrooms?" I asked, looking him right in the eye.

"Huh?" he replied, nose crinkled, disgust creeping into his face.

"Listen," I said. "Personally, I can't stand 'em. They look funny, sometimes they smell funny and, in fact, they are a type of fungus!"

Angelo relaxed the nose and lifted his eyebrows. Clearly he was in agreement. His mom, on the other hand, started eyeing me suspiciously.

"But here's the problem," I continued. "Everyone I know thinks they're just great! Really, my mom, my sister, my husband…they all think I'm really missing out. I don't know, but I'm willing to make a deal with you. I bet I like mushrooms even less than you, but I also bet that neither you nor I have ever tried them. I sure haven't, have you?"

Angelo thought a minute and shook his head. He was ready to admit he hadn't really tried mushrooms before.

So we struck a deal. Angelo and I would both make an honest attempt to try mushrooms sometime before our next meeting. We agreed that there were no promises, no guarantees, but that we would both give it our best shot. If one of us tried mushrooms, the other would have to live up to the agreement and try them too. A handshake confirmed the deal as I turned to Angelo's mom to discuss strategies to make food appealing to the picky eater.

Later that week, my husband Mike and I were out for dinner when I told him laughingly about the bet.

"Well," laughed Mike, "tonight is a great time to try mushrooms then…how convenient that the dish I ordered has mushrooms in it!"

I gasped realizing that I was in trouble. But remembering Angelo, I allowed Mike to ease one onto my plate. Of course I wasn't getting off easy. It was one of those big brown floppy kinds that looked half alive, as if it was just swiped off the forest's floor. I moved it around on my plate as long as possible, until the guilt was getting to me and, quite frankly, there was nowhere to hide. Holding my nose and breath, I gently lifted the mushroom to my lips and…dropped it back to the plate. Mike's loving glance was tainted with mockery and disbelief.

"Can't do it, can you?" he laughed, genuinely unaware of my agony.

"Listen," I said. "What are the chances, after this long?"

We finished our meal and headed home. I quickly forgot the incident until a couple of weeks later when Angelo and his family arrived for his baby sister's checkup. I should have known something was up when Angelo rushed into the room, clearly excited about the visit. Angelo's brothers rushed to my side, announcing that there was some important news to share. I turned to Angelo.

"So, Angelo, how's your baby sister doing?"

"Oh she's fine Dr Ganju, but I have something important to tell you!"

As it turned out, a few nights before, their family had gone out for dinner to a Chinese restaurant. One of the dishes had mushrooms in it and, of his own accord, with the whole family bearing witness, Angelo ate a mushroom!

"No," I gasped, "You didn't!" In fact, I felt a little queasy myself suddenly recalling the mushroom I had rejected. I regained my composure and, genuinely curious, asked what it was like.

"Do you know what, Dr Ganju? At first I was nervous, but then I really wanted to try it, and it was good!"

Somewhat in disbelief, I shifted my glance to his mother. Beaming, she offered confirmation.

"What's more, he ate a couple of mushrooms and then even tried a green bean!"

I looked down to the floor. My heart flooded with emotion—pride for Angelo about conquering his fears, sadness for myself, still so stunted and unable to appreciate the mushroom. Angelo, suddenly sensing my apprehension, took on a wisdom much beyond his years. He crossed the room to my side, placed his hand on my arm, and said gently, "Don't worry, Dr Ganju. If you just try them, I'll bet you will like them too!"

Ameeta Ganju, MD
Chicago, IL

Chapter 4

The Irrepressible Logic of Children

Part I

I was making rounds and stopped to say hello to a 5½-year-old boy who had been in the hospital for about 10 days recovering from complications of a ruptured appendix. There were many "get well" cards all over the room and, after saying hello to him and inquiring about how he was doing, I asked if I could read some of the cards. He said, "OK." Several of these were from classmates; one of them asked, "Why are you in the hospital? Are you having a baby?"

Mohsen Ziai, MD
Falls Church, VA

℘

I was trying very hard to get a 4-year-old boy to do some exercises one day. All I wanted was for him to jump up and down to see if the irregularity of his heartbeat would go away. That is, after all, how 4-year-old boys spend their lives. Should be easy, shouldn't it? But no, in no way would he do that. So I asked him to sit up, lie down, sit up, lie down. After about 4 times, he looked me in the eye and said, "Can't you make up your mind?!!"

Chloe G. Alexson, MD
Rochester, NY

Recently, after examining a young man and diagnosing him with streptococcal pharyngitis, we discussed the options of obtaining a Bicillin injection for treatment. The patient looked at me very seriously and said, "I don't want to insult you, but I would like to see your diploma. We walked back to my office, where he inspected my diploma very carefully without saying a word. The patient walked back to the exam room, shaking his head, and got back on the table and said, "Well, it looked pretty legitimate to me. I guess we will have to go ahead and do it."

Stephen P. Combs, MD
Gray, TN

℘

I have a habit of addressing the mothers accompanying children as "Mom." One day, I entered the examining room to take a look at a 4-year-old and asked, "How is Scott, Mom?"

"Oh, he has a runny nose and an earache."

All of a sudden, Scott became somewhat concerned and, with a curious look, he asked his mother, "Are you his mom too, Mom?"

There was a pause for a few seconds, and then the mother and I burst out in laughter. How innocent a child's world can be!

Amar Dave, MD
Ottowa, IL

My 5-year-old grandson was visiting us and he suddenly asked when his mother was going to pick him up. I answered, "In about twenty minutes."

He then told me that 100 is greater than 20 and infinity is greater than 100. I asked, "What is infinity?"

He said, "It is a part of God."

I asked, "Who told you that?"

He answered, "No one. I figured it out myself."

I now find it a bit difficult to carry on a conversation with him!

Neal McNabb, MD
Honeoye Falls, NY

✒

During a physical examination on a young boy I was urging him to breathe in, breathe out, breathe in, breathe out. A concerned child looked up at me and said, "How else could I breathe?"

Mary Ellen Avery, MD
Boston, MA

✒

Growing up on a farm, 4-year-old Patrick was very familiar with planting and growing vegetables and trees. One morning he came running into the kitchen and announced with some fear in his eyes, "Mother, I just swallowed a cherry pit. If I now eat some soil and fertilizer will a cherry tree grow out of my head?"

Claus Helbing, MD
Annandale, VA

An 8-year-old girl arrived in my office for her first visit. I started the chart by asking her questions about her name, her address, and her phone number. The discussion continued as follows:

Doctor: "What is your birthday?"
Young girl: "August 24th."
Doctor: "What year?"
Young girl: "Every year!"

Solomon J. Cohen, MD
New York, NY

℘

When my son was 4 years old, he was helping me prepare dinner. He wanted to help me with cutting up some carrots. Not wanting him to use the knife, I told him he couldn't help me with the carrots until he was bigger. Taking me very literally, he proceeded to climb on a chair and said, "I'm bigger now Mommy!"

Toby Jacobowitz, MD
Ann Arbor, MI

℘

Two 8-year-old girls met after school to talk about their upcoming spring break.

"Why don't you come to the beach with me and my family?" one of them asked.

"I'd like to," said her friend, "but I wet the bed at night so I'm nervous about taking trips with my friends."

"How often do you wet the bed?" the first girl asked.

"About once a week."

"That's simple," her friend answered. "Just wet your bed the night before we leave."

Howard J. Bennett, MD
Washington, DC

✆

My wife had suffered through a case of kidney stones, and our 4-year-old son was understandably concerned about his mother. A few days after the episode he announced that he was confused, "How can Mommy have *kid*ney stones? Shouldn't kids only have them?"

Robert S. Bahadori, MD
Fairfax, VA

✆

As I walked into an examining room one afternoon for a well-baby exam, I was greeted by a mother breastfeeding her 2-month-old infant. The baby's sibling, 3 years old, was busy watching the feeding and talking with her mother. After greeting the older child and her mother, I started to discuss the breastfeeding and how things were going when the very attentive 3-year-old offered her opinion. She stated that she was going to breastfeed her child when she got older, just like Mommy, but added that one side would be for milk and the other for orange juice! Needless to say the mother and I were in stitches the rest of the exam, and the story quickly spread throughout my office to the delight of all of the staff.

Delosa Young, MD
Rockville, MD

Chapter 5

Here Comes Trouble!

The 5-year-old girl was very unhappy about having to come for her checkup. Being weighed in was annoying, and she did not like having her height measured. Taking her blood pressure was very difficult, having to listen for it over her complaining. By the time her vision was being checked, her yelling could be heard throughout the office as she voiced her objections ever more loudly about what was being done. Finally, the nurse gave her a cup and explained that she wanted her to pee in it. That was the last straw. She looked at it incredulously and shouted out disbelievingly, "You expect me to sit on that?"

Jon Matthew Farber, MD
Alexandria, VA

℘

I had a call from a mother who said her child had been cut on barnacles. Because I was practicing in Denver, 1,000 miles from the nearest ocean, I couldn't figure out how this could have happened. It turned out the child was swimming around a pier in Southern California and had been scratched on a cluster of barnacles. The mother immediately arranged for a flight back to Denver. We saw the child on an emergency basis and carefully applied a Band-Aid.

James E. Strain, MD
Denver, CO

It was 5:30 pm and we were about to close when the call came from the local hospital. The emergency department physician was quite concerned. A 14-year-old boy had fainted in school and was brought to the emergency department by ambulance. They needed my advice. As seizures and cardiac events went through my mind, I asked for more history, and the other physician began. Today was the day they showed the film *The Miracle of Life* in family life class. The film discussed conception and delivery of a newborn. I interrupted and said, "You're not going to tell me that as the baby exited the birth canal, Forrest fainted?"

"That is exactly what happened," he replied. He reported that Forrest was feeling just fine now, and the CBC, blood electrolytes, CAT scan, and skull film were all normal. "What do you want to do with the patient?" he asked.

"Send him home, keep him out of a medical field, don't make him finish watching the film, and don't ex-pect him to be of any help during any of his future wife's deliveries," was my medical advice.

Carl A. Salsbury, MD
Falls Church, VA

It was a busy but quiet morning in the office, when suddenly there was a loud screaming commotion in the waiting room. My receptionist rapidly ushered 2 police-men and a totally hysterical young mother and her baby into a recently vacated waiting room. I left the patient I had been examining, expecting to see something terrible.

After a few minutes, we had quieted the mother and asked what was wrong. The baby, a robust, active, 4-month-old lay smiling on the table. The mother finally told us that the baby's penis had fallen off. "It was there earlier this morning, but when I changed his diaper later, it was gone. It fell off. I looked all over the room, even under the radiator, but couldn't find it." She had no car, so she called the police to bring her to the office.

I quietly unpinned the diaper, pressed down on the large pre-pubic fat pad, exposing the "hidden" penis. The sobbing mother now cried with joy. After I explained to her what had happened, she left with the 2 quite relieved policemen. We then had a good laugh. Later, when we found out that even the police were on their hands and knees looking for the penis that had "fallen off," we had another good laugh.

David Annunziato, MD
East Meadow, NY

✄

Thursday, July 9, was just a bad day for 5-year-old Francine. She arrived at her pediatrician's office bewildered, angry, and resistant. Even with my best approach, a little nonthreatening conversation while she sat on her mother's lap, I knew we were in for a confrontation when she refused to sit on the examining table or take off her clothes and put on a pretty gown for her yearly exam.

Her mother, thoroughly embarrassed by this behavior, was unsuccessful in breaking her resistance. We held her for the ear and nose exam, pried open her mouth, and checked her heart, lungs, and abdomen while she tightly gripped her clothes. Not getting too far with the details of her examination, we ended it but only after she finalized her anger by throwing her sock at the doctor.

Mom took this behavior badly and called Dad on her cell phone to report the day's events and charged him with a serious father-daughter talk as soon as he arrived home. When Dad arrived from work that evening, he found Francine sitting in a chair, eyes downcast, and unwilling to speak. On his way home, he had decided that the seriousness of Francine's misbehavior called for something more than the usual restrictions and scolding. So, to emphasize his displeasure, he calmly, yet firmly, instructed Francine to report to the master bedroom where he and her mom would discuss the matter with her in private. With an air of legal formality, he told Francine to sit on the end of the bed and then asked her mom to retell the story of the visit to the doctor. Dad stood watching Francine, her eyes still downcast, as they both listened to Mom's indictment.

When Mom was finished, Dad looked at Francine with an expression of disappointment and disbelief as he began his carefully planned lecture by slowly, and with great seriousness, asking a question, "Francine, have you gone off the deep end?"

Francine raised her eyes and responded, somewhat confused, still scared, but with complete sincerity, "But Daddy, I didn't even get to go to the pool today!"

Peter Nachajski, MD
Alexandria, VA

The new sheriff of a local town is a very nice woman with 2 small children. I had completed exams of both of her children, and we needed to prick their fingers to get some blood. The 6-year-old screamed loudly enough to damage the 2 sets of ears in the next exam room. "Make her stop," he yelled repeatedly.

His mom said that we needed to do the blood test and she couldn't make the nurse stop. With tears in his eyes he pleaded, "But Mom, you're the sheriff."

Carl A. Salsbury, MD
Falls Church, VA

☙

During a recent clinic visit, I was evaluating a child from Kosovo who recently immigrated to the United States. A teenaged cousin of the patient was serving as translator during the visit. In the middle of the visit, the receptionist announced over the speaker that the owner of a green car had left its lights on. I asked the family if they had a green car. I heard the teenager talk to the adult uncle in their native language. Then, the father pulled out his wallet and was searching for something, but seemed worried and upset that he couldn't find it.

When I asked him what was wrong, he said, "We can't find our Green Card."

I told him that he didn't need it to see me in the clinic and burst into laughter!

Majdi M. Abu-Salih, MD
Hartford, WI

When I was a resident at a hospital in New York City in the early 1950s, I was on duty one night when a 3-year-old boy was admitted to my floor. His mother had brought him to the emergency department because he was irritable and felt feverish. The nurse in the emergency department placed him on the examining table and inserted a thermometer in his rectum, holding him prone with one hand. He suddenly wiggled free and sat upright. The thermometer slid all the way in and could not be retrieved despite single-digit efforts to slide it out. He was admitted for proctoscopy for fear the thermometer might break and perforate his rectum. I took him into the examining room and decided to try a double-digit extraction in the hope of avoiding anesthesia and proctoscopy.

I was successful and turned to his mother triumphantly holding the thermometer aloft and said, "Everything is all right. You can take him home."

Her response was, "So, what's his temperature?"

Robert Hoekelman, MD
Rochester, NY

I was just trying to be a nice guy, but they often do finish last. My oldest was in the second grade, and I offered to take the class to the hospital. The class had more than 40 children, so we split it in half. As we toured the nursery, I pointed out a premature baby weighing about 4 pounds. We next headed to the lab, and the director spoke about medical laboratories and various lab tests they can do.

She then asked if the children would like to see a unit of blood. They shouted, "Yes," and she pulled out a bag of blood.

As she pointed out the difference between the layers of red and white cells, Eddie did a 360-degree turn and fell flat on his face onto his wire-rim glasses, thereby lacerating his face. Eddie was now out cold in a faint with blood dripping about his face. Martin was next and slumped to the floor. Two more followed.

I was now on my knees trying to stem Eddie's blood flow and glanced over at the first-year second grade teacher who looked very pale and shaky. As we quickly hid the bag of blood and began to hurriedly vacate the laboratory, I picked up the revived Eddie to take him to the emergency department for necessary sutures. I said, "Eddie, tell your friends that you are OK."

Eddie just lay limply in my arms with his tongue hanging out, and the other children stared pale and open mouthed. I repeated, "Eddie, tell everyone you're OK." Nothing.

Finally I said, "Boys and girls, Eddie is just fine," and headed downstairs to the emergency department, where I met a very aggravated mother.

A week later the school called, thanked me for my field trip, and asked when I would be able to take the second half of that grade. It has been 17 years now, and I guess they are still waiting.

Carl A. Salsbury, MD
Falls Church, VA

A nonresponsive, strapping, 16-year-old male was rushed into the emergency department. Vigorous stimulation, including a sternal rub applied with the full strength of the examiner, failed to elicit a response. His friend explained this alarming condition as a reaction to a bee sting. About 30 minutes ago, they were "hanging out" in a park. When stung, the patient had exclaimed he had always been allergic to bee stings and then gradually had stopped responding.

Further quick physical examination revealed an upper extremity lesion (3 cm in diameter) consistent with an insect sting, otherwise normal skin, normal vital signs, normal respiratory pattern, and a normal lung exam.

With respiratory and cardiovascular systems apparently intact, a more detailed examination was performed. There was no evidence of head trauma; neck was supple; and neurologic examination, with the exception of mental status, was also normal.

While neurology was paged and the relative merits of lumbar puncture, magnetic resonance imaging, and computerized axial tomography were debated by other doctors, a contemplative pediatrician repeatedly raised the patient's arm a short distance above the young man's face and dropped it. After about 10 repetitions, the young man's hand started missing his face.

At this point, the pensive pediatrician gently informed the young man of the many indications that he was doing very well indeed—his breathing, his heartbeat, his blood pressure—all this surely pointed to a steady recovery. After repeating this reassurance, the young man was informed that pretty soon he'd be ready to squeeze the examiner's hand. And then, before long, he'd be able to squeeze harder and harder.

Fifteen minutes later, while sitting up and chatting engagingly with the pediatrician, the young man revealed that his family conviction in bee sting allergy was based on a badly swollen hand at age 3 years. Also, he had recently seen the Hollywood hit *Arachnophobia*. The young man agreed with the pediatrician—it was a pretty scary movie.

Kenneth M. McConnochie, MD
Rochester, NY

☙

When I was a resident, a family arrived in the emergency department and asked me to examine their child, who allegedly had been acting strangely fatigued and intermittently feverish. After examining her thoroughly, I admitted that I could find nothing other than a benign heart murmur. They immediately smiled, perked up, and said, "Fine, now we'll bring in the child who is really sick; we were just testing you."

Samuel L. Katz, MD
Durham, NC

One Sunday, late at night, I examined a patient with abdominal pain in my office. The child did not have any sign of an acute abdomen, and I felt that she had some spasm. I wrote a prescription for the father to have filled. The next day the father returned to the office with the prescription in hand. He told me he was not able to find an "all-night drugstore" last night, the child got better, therefore, he was returning the prescription and requested his money back for the visit!!!

S. Mahallati, MD
Grasonville, MD

Chapter 6

Heartwarming Tales
Part I

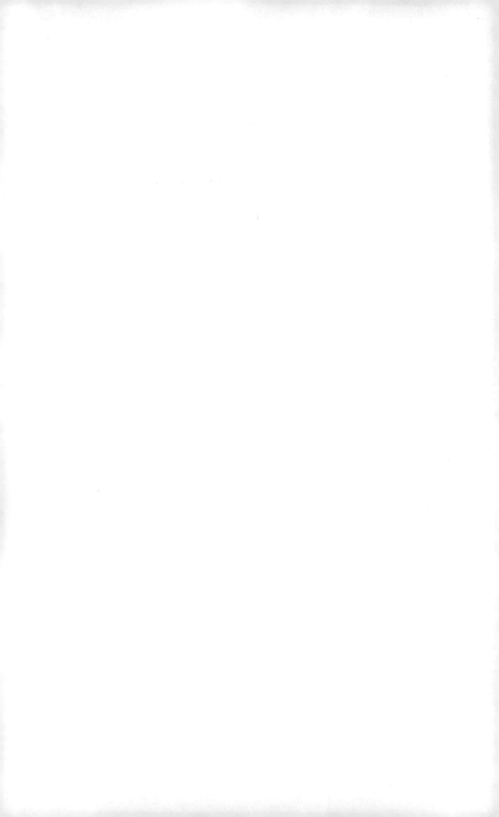

When I was a pediatric intern in Rochester, NY, one of my frequent tasks was to draw blood and place an intravenous line in oncology patients who were frequently admitted for chemotherapy or fevers with neutropenia (low white blood cell count). A little boy named Jack came in one day for one of many admissions, and was unusually cheerful. Pleased not to be confronted with a crying and unhappy child, I gathered my syringes, needles, tape, blood tubes, and IV fluid and went to his bedside. As I placed my equipment at his side, he suddenly whipped out his hands and squirted me with 60 cc of water from a big syringe, right in the face. I was speechless, but quickly dissolved in laughter as we exchanged looks; mine of shock, his of mirth.

Though I later sadly cared for Jack as he lay dying of complications of his chemotherapy, I will never forget him or the gift he gave me that day in the emergency department.

Steve Keller, MD
Falls Church, VA

✄

A 7-year-old boy was diagnosed with cancer. The mother, convinced that the child would be teased because of his baldness, did not want to send him to school. Finally, the oncology team convinced her that attending school was in her child's best interest.

School began at 8:30 am. By 9:00 am the parent could no longer stand the tension. Convinced that something bad had surely occurred, she hurried to the school. The teacher met her outside the classroom and assured her that there was no problem. Indeed, the teacher said that the child was becoming financially well off.

"How can that be?" asked the mother.

"He is charging his classmates ten cents each to go into a dark room where he takes off his wig and lets them rub his bald head!"

Bruce M. Camitta, MD
Milwaukee, WI

✆

A lesson in "heart" is my 10-year-old daughter, Sarah, who was born with a muscle missing in her foot and wears a brace all the time. She came home one beautiful spring day to tell me she had competed in "field day"— that's where they have lots of races and other competitive events.

Because of her leg support, my mind raced as I tried to think of encouragement for my Sarah, things I could say to her about not letting this get her down, but before I could get a word out she said, "Daddy, I won two of the races!"

I couldn't believe it! And then Sarah said, "I had an advantage."

Ah. I knew it. I thought she must have been given a head start…some kind of physical advantage. But again, before I could say anything, she said, "Daddy, I didn't get a head start…my advantage was I had to try harder!"

Jim Caffee, MD
Fresno, CA

Quite a few years ago, we were taking care of a 14-year-old boy who had had major problems in surgery, including serious bleeding with possible neurologic consequences. He was making a long, slow but steady recovery. I was at his bedside when one of the surgical residents came by and asked him if any of the doctors had removed some of his stitches. The conversation follows.

"Bobby, did one of the doctors come by and take out some of your stitches?"

"I don't know."

"Bobby, did one of the other doctors take out every other one of the stitches we put in to close your incision?"

"I don't know."

"Bobby" (said very slowly and distinctly with some exasperation), "you're fourteen years old. Tell me if one of the doctors took out some of your stitches."

"Gee, Doc, don't ask me. I'm the one with the short-term memory loss."

Chloe G. Alexson, MD
Rochester, NY

✆

This occurred while I was in pediatric training. I was a senior resident in charge of one of our pediatric wings with surgical patients of various ages. We were assigned several children and rounded every morning and at sign-off.

One patient that brings back certain memories was a young girl who had a giant hemangioma of her right leg. This was quite extensive; so much so that surgery was not an option at that time. Her outlook always was positive, and she had a smile to top all.

Every morning, for some reason, I would wind up playing tic-tac-toe with her. This was a ritual that was repeated every day. To her delight, she was always there waiting, not complaining of an ailment that would probably do her in. And every morning, wouldn't you know, that smile would beat me.

This ritual went on for quite a while. Always she would wonder when Dr Larry would drop in. As you can imagine, when I was transferred to another rotation, it was not easy. One morning, the parents called me in, probably to see me get beaten again, but also to win a smile from their daughter. After the big match, the mother gave me a key chain. Engraved on one side was a tic-tac-toe symbol and inscribed on the other side was: "Hope you win them all." To date, I still have that key ring; and I hope that she won them all too.

A. Larry Miller, MD
Vienna, VA

✄

Three-year-old Aaron's grandfather died recently. He was proud of his balloon, which was given to him in a restaurant. As he was leaving the restaurant with his family, the balloon got away, flying into the sky. His mother remarked, "Oh Aaron, what a pity that the balloon is flying off." Aaron replied without any regrets, "It's all right, Mom, it's going to Grandpa."

Claus Helbing, MD
Annandale, VA

In the days before modern techniques, children needing intravenous antibiotics for 6 to 8 weeks had to struggle by with peripheral IVs. One such child, a very engaging 18-month-old boy with osteomyelitis (infection of the bones), was rapidly running out of sites. Into the treatment room went the "torture team," the RN and I, and the victim. He was one of those children who cried when hurt, sobbed in between times, but never moved the extremity being stuck. He was being exceptionally good; I was failing miserably. Finally, after the umpteenth unsuccessful attempt, we were all sweating, upset, and in need of a break. We stopped, removed the tourniquet, and let him sit up. Still sobbing, he reached over to the stack of as yet unopened IVs and handed me the next one.

Feeling like a complete slime, I got it into a much used and abused vein in the arm. Believe it or not, it lasted for more than 2 weeks!

Peter D. Grundl, MD
Falls Church, VA

As a young attending, I cared for a teenager with severe heart failure. I was supporting him during a thoracentesis (when a needle is put into the chest to draw fluid). He looked up and said, "You smell so good." I wasn't wearing any perfume.

Jacqueline A. Noonan, MD
Lexington, KY

A 9-year-old girl was in the hospital with a chylothorax, a complication following repair of pulmonic stenosis (a partial obstruction of the conduit from the heart to the lungs). She was on a no-fat diet that she found quite difficult to follow. We all felt sorry for her, but she made our lives difficult constantly trying to bargain for something that would taste better. All of a sudden her complaints stopped and she spent the rest of the time having baked potatoes with strawberry jam 3 times a day—not really all that bad when you try it.

Chloe G. Alexson, MD
Rochester, NY

Chapter 7

Kids Say the Darndest Things
Part II

A 12-year-old boy came to the office with fever and sore throat after a sporting event. When I had finished the examination, he asked if I would continue to be his pediatrician for a long time.

I told him, "You are one of my favorite patients. I'll continue to see you as long as I am in practice."

He looked at me in puzzlement and asked, "Dr Chusuei, are you still practicing to be a doctor?"

Richard V. Chusuei, MD
McLean, VA

✆

I was in the process of doing a complete sports history and physical for a 16-year-old high school football player. When I asked him, "Are you allergic to grass?" he looked at me, then turned his head so slightly and quietly murmured, "Oh Doc, I hardly ever use it."

Gary M. Gorlick, MD
Los Angeles, CA

✆

I had laryngitis and after performing a physical examination on a 4-year-old boy named Danny, I started to discuss his growth and development with the mother. When Danny heard my hoarse voice, he said, "Dr Russo, now I can check you. I got a new doctor's kit for my birthday."

Voja Russo, MD
Great Falls, VA

My patient was 4 years old when it was time to send him for ear tubes. On a subsequent visit to my office, his mother told me that at his visit with the ENT, he said to the specialist, "You're not a doctor 'cause only girls are doctors!"

Lynne Ellis, MD
St Petersburg, FL

✆

A long time ago my 3-year-old granddaughter and I were discussing the day she was born. She asked me where I had been when she was born, and I replied that I was unable to be at her birth but her grandmother had traveled to be at the delivery and had given me the good news of her healthy arrival as soon as she was born.

My granddaughter thought for a moment and then asked, "Then where was I when *you* were born?"

Mohsen Ziai, MD
Falls Church, VA

✆

I asked a 7-year-old girl, who was clinging to her mother and had been brought in because of pain in the tummy, "Do you have abdominal pains now?"

The girl regarded me for a moment, then looked at her mother, and in all honesty asked, "Mom, do I have abdominal pain?"

John G. Bitar, MD
McLean, VA

One day I saw a 4-year-old girl with pain on urination who had a normal urinalysis and a mildly red introitus. When I told the mom that her daughter's urethra was irritated, the girl said, "It's not *your* rethra, it's *my* rethra!"

Howard J. Bennett, MD
Washington, DC

♋

I was examining a 6-year-old boy and noticed he had a right lower quadrant scar from an appendectomy. I asked him when he'd had his appendix taken out. He told me that it was on the Fourth of July and, incidentally, his hospital room had a view overlooking the harbor where the fireworks are set off. I commented on how that must have been so exciting to see. Then he said to me, "Do you know where I was when the fireworks were going off?" I looked at him, puzzled.
"In the operating room!" was his reply.

Kenneth Colmer, MD
South Yarmouth, MA

♋

My dad, at age 75, had developed laryngeal carcinoma, and in those days only a laryngectomy held hope of a total cure. He was walking down the hall in my office, and garrulous as he was, he was speaking to everyone. I was in a room examining a 4-year-old boy. As he overheard my dad talking through his vibrator, the boy's eyes became as big as saucers and he said, "There's a robot out there."

Robert Herndon, MD
Chickasha, OK

℘

Recently, working alongside our state health department to improve immunization rates, we held an event to publicize the new immunization effort. We were delighted when our state's first lady, Mrs Barbara Richardson, took on the job of honorary chair of our effort and said she would come. She then invited 2 of her friends, Betty Bumpers (former first lady of Arkansas) and Rosalyn Carter, both of whom have been very active in working for improved immunization rates throughout the country. We were very excited by their coming to join us.

I thought that perhaps that morning my 14-year-old patient might want to wait around afterward to meet Mrs Carter, Mrs Bumpers, and Mrs Richardson. So I asked her, "Mary, do you know who Rosalyn Carter is?"

"No," she said thoughtfully.

"Well," I returned, "do you know who Jimmy Carter is?"

"Sure. He was a member of a rock group, right?"

Lance A. Chilton, MD
Albuquerque, NM

One of my 3-year-old female patients was in the exam room waiting for me. Her mother was keeping her occupied by explaining the drawing of the circulatory system that was hanging on the wall. The last thing she seems to have remembered was the description of the ventricles. So, when I came into the room, she excitedly asked, "Are you going to listen to my testicles?" She has never lived it down.

Kelly Bruce Lobley, MD
Spring, TX

℘

Young children have the usually endearing, sometimes embarrassing, quality of uttering uninhibited comments about people, places, and things. I was in the midst of a physical examination on a 5-year-old in our Diagnostic Referral Clinic at Johns Hopkins a few years back when the youngster asked innocently if I were a vampire. Thinking that he was envisioning an upcoming venipuncture, I asked how he knew. "Your teeth," he replied, commenting on my prominent canines!

Walter W. Tunnessen, Jr, MD
Chapel Hill, NC

One of my new nurses was getting a detailed history, and knowing that I insisted on having it filled out completely, she was intent on getting it just right.

She read the blank history sheet and asked, "Name?" She recorded that information. Then she asked, "Address?" and wrote that down. Without looking up, she said, "Sex?"

The young man answered, "No my parents won't let me."

Ask for it, you get it.

Claude A. Frazier, MD
Asheville, NC

✆

"Dr Hertz" is a difficult name for a pediatrician to have because kids take things so literally. One young patient of mine, on hearing from his mom that he was going to see Dr Hertz, said thoughtfully, "Doctor hurts? Jesus make her all better."

Gail S. Hertz, MD
York, PA

✆

One of my little patients was anxious to begin kindergarten. Finally, one day he inquired of his father, "Daddy when can I go to "Kendig garten"?

Edwin Lawrence Kendig, Jr, MD
Richmond, VA

Currently I am a developmental pediatrician. As part of my evaluation I routinely throw a ball back and forth with my patients. One of my patients later asked his primary physician why he did not play ball with him like Dr Nussbaum does.

Dan Nussbaum, MD
Brockport, NY

✆

When my daughter was at her 4-year checkup, the doctor was impressed by her command of the language. He decided to begin asking her the 5-year-old developmental questions. At one point, he asked her what you do at the lake. She looked up at him very seriously, scrunched up her nose and said, "Oh that is a very long story!"

We both laughed, but she continued to say, "You don't have time for it, your patients are waiting."

Madhu Henry, MD
Washington, DC

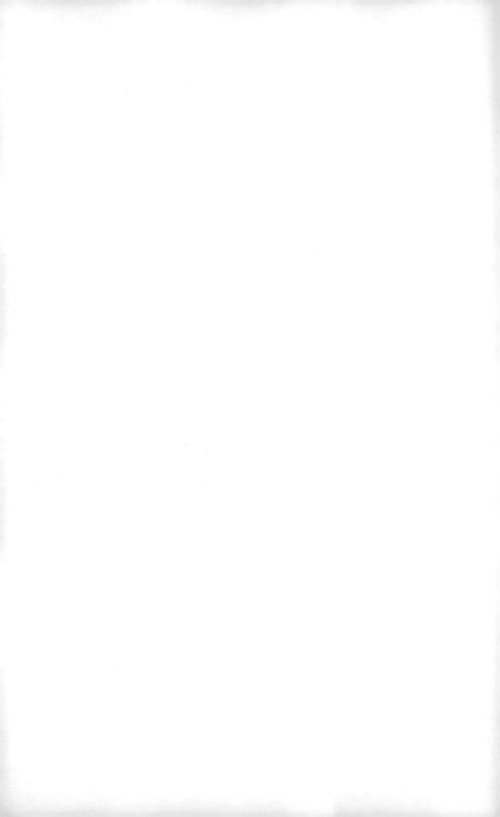

Chapter 8

Kids *Do* the Darndest Things

A young boy came into the office dressed in a Superman costume and was on the exam table while I chatted with his mother. As I turned to address him, he grabbed my tie and yelled, "Geronimo!" and swung off the table. Needless to say I had sore neck muscles for several days.

Marvin Tabb, MD
Silver Spring, MD

✺

A 5-year-old girl came to the clinic with the chief complaint of "something up the nose." The something turned out to be a button that was rather far up the nares (nasal openings) and required some time and an alligator forceps to extract. The child was remarkably good about the whole procedure, although it must have been rather uncomfortable. The mother, on the other hand, was mortified.

As I was reassuring her that kids do these things, the little girl piped up, "I'm going to put a bigger one up there next time!"

Peter D. Grundl, MD
Falls Church, VA

✺

I had just finished a routine physical examination on one of my favorite patients, a bright, happy 10-year-old, when I asked, "Do you have a hobby, Gerald?"

He said, "Yes, herpetology."

I asked, "You collect snakes?"

"Yes," he said.

I told him that I had a phobia for snakes. Thereafter, whenever he or his brothers came to the office, he would produce a snake from his pocket and chase me around the office. At one visit, his mother and I convinced him to promise he would never do it again. A few months later, after a visit, he confronted me with a snake from one of his pockets.

When I recovered and reminded him of his promise, he responded, "I made that promise with a mental reservation."

David Annunziato, MD
East Meadow, NY

✺

On finishing my exam on a most pleasant and polite 5-year-old boy, I pulled from my pocket, as usual, a couple of lollipops and gave them to him as a reward for his cooperation. He looked at me for a moment, then put his hand in his pocket, searched for a while, and pulled out a dime, paying for his lollipops!

John G. Bitar, MD
McLean, VA

✺

I remember the phone ringing one morning when I was eager to get started. Paul's mother was distressed. He would eat nothing but tuna fish morning, noon, and night. It was easy to allay her fears. Our son, Steve, was at that moment eating his (at least) 72nd consecutive tuna fish breakfast.

Henry M. Seidel, MD
Baltimore, MD

※

The patient's ear was bruised and she denied any accident. Her parents were not aware of any fall and were concerned that the bruising was due to a bleeding disorder. The 5-year-old was ready with the explanation. "My daddy can play the piano by ear, and so can I."

Carl A. Salsbury, MD
Falls Church, VA

※

I was going through the Denver Developmental Screening Test with a 3½-year-old boy. I asked him if he could stand on one foot. He nodded his head and walked over and stood on my right foot.

Thomas B. Newman, MD
San Francisco, CA

※

After falling at school, an 8-year-old girl came to my office. Her distal left forearm was swollen, mildly deformed, and exquisitely tender. I told her mother that it was likely it was fractured based on my exam. The mother suggested that it might be only sprained.

"No, it's likely broken," I reiterated. "It looks like it, sounds like it, and smells like it."

At which point, the young lady raised her newly splinted arm to her nose and sniffed.

She turned out to have a buckle fracture of the distal ulna.

Wanda Lo, MD
San Luis Obispo, CA

❧

On being presented with a "draw-a-person" test sometime in the early 1970s, an 8-year-old drew a very strange figure: a cylinder with a rounded top and little feet protruding from the bottom. It had no eyes, ears, nose, or mouth, just dials and knobs. And it had no arms or hands. Before concluding that this child was psychotic or developmentally disabled, I asked my own 8-year-old to interpret the drawing. He said, "Dad, you need to go to the movies. That drawing is of R2D2 from *Star Wars!*"

I then asked my patient what he meant to draw and was politely informed R2D2...of course!

Phil Davidson, MD
Rochester, NY

❧

A mother brought her 2-year-old daughter into the office right after Thanksgiving because "her eye smells." I leaned over the child and, sure enough, there was a foul odor coming from the vicinity of her right eye. On more careful scrutiny, I noticed a thick discharge coming from her right nostril. After a little suctioning, it was evident that there was a small black object in the middle of the puddle of pus in the right nostril. With a forceps I extracted a whole clove. On seeing it, the mother gasped, "Oh my goodness…the Easter ham!" That was a well-seasoned clove.

Lawrence F. Nazarian, MD
Rochester, NY

✠

The mother of a 4-year-old boy told me her child was fascinated by the trash man on his weekly rounds. He would sit on the front porch the day of the pickup, patiently waiting for the trash man to appear. For his fourth birthday his mother gave him a trash can with the appropriate amount of trash. He was thrilled.

James E. Strain, MD
Denver, CO

✠

Recently a young lady came in complaining of ear pain. I asked her what was wrong with her ear, and she said she had gravel in her ear. On exam, sure enough she had gravel lodged in both canals. I asked her why she had gravel, and she stated that it was her rock collection. After multiple attempts to remove the small rocks, I put them in a small container for her. The child looked up and said, "Boy, doctors are so smart. That is much easier than carrying those rocks around in my head."

Stephen P. Combs, MD
Gray, TN

✆

To help young children relax during office visits, I find bunnies and other animals "hiding" in their ears. After a recent well-child visit, a mother took her 2-year-old daughter to a restaurant for lunch. Halfway through the meal, the mom noticed that her daughter was trying to put a piece of lettuce in her ear. When asked what she was doing, the little girl replied, "I'm feeding the bunny."

Howard J. Bennett, MD
Washington, DC

✆

I was performing a neurologic exam on a 10-year-old boy with possible Asperger disorder, whose mother warned me that he interpreted things very literally.

After ascertaining that he knew how to identify right and left on me when I was facing him, I asked him to match my finger movements, right hand to right hand, and left to left, instructing him, "Do what I do."

I touched my right thumb and index finger and so did he. I touched my left thumb and fifth finger—he matched me. My nose was running—he matched me sniff for sniff.

Smiling, I moved on to what I thought was a task with more concrete instructions. "Come over here and hop on one foot," I said.

He obediently hopped up and down on my foot. "No, no," I said, "pick up one of your feet and hop up and down."

He did—on my foot.

His complete befuddlement over the laughter of his mother and me only helped to confirm the diagnosis.

Stephen Sulkes, MD
Rochester, NY

✄

Sometimes we forget how literal and concrete kids can be. Example: I told a child to get ready and jump up on my examining table so that I could examine him. Imagine my surprise when he climbed onto the examining table and began to jump up and down, up and down!

Andrea Weaver, MD
Herndon, VA

✄

It was a hot July day when my wife commented that our son's teeth looked a bit yellow. She asked if he was brushing daily, and he replied that he had lost his toothbrush. She asked when this happened, and he smiled a yellow smile and said, "May."

Carl A. Salsbury, MD
Falls Church, VA

Little Molly told her mother matter-of-factly, "A piece of wood just fell out of my ear."

Her mother asked her, "What did you do with it?"

"I threw it away," she replied, not much concerned. Molly had ventilation tubes placed because of frequent ear infections and they were ready to come out.

Claus Helbing, MD
Annandale, VA

✌

One day I was getting a weight on a young boy about 6 or 7 years old. When he stood on the scale, I noticed he had gained quite a bit of weight. I jokingly asked, "What do you have, some rocks in your pockets?"

He quickly replied, "Yeah! I was saving them for my rock collection!"

He proceeded to pull out handfuls of rocks from each of his pants pockets. Needless to say, we laughed all day.

Diane Dubinsky, MD
Fairfax, VA

Chapter 9

The Blooper Reel

The 3-year-old was screaming, and I was trying to explain how often the medication was needed and the potential side effects. Michael continued screaming, and I was sure that the mother was getting less than half of my discussion. She repeatedly asked the child to calm down, and he continued screaming. Finally she lost it and, in a very stern tone, said, "Michael, be quiet! I can't hear the doctor. Now calm down! What are you crying about anyway?" Between sobs, Michael blurted, "Dr Salsbury's chair is on my foot."

Carl A. Salsbury, MD
Falls Church, VA

☏

A young boy named Charlie and his father came into the emergency department because Charlie had a bad rash. The intern on call wanted a consult with the pediatric resident, so I was called. I inquired what the child ate, and the only change in diet was cantaloupe. Being a French-speaking Belgian, I thought "cantaloupe" was the English translation of "antelope," so I was puzzled how my patient ate that in the summer. I asked the father if he had shot it, if he hunts a lot, if he used many bullets to kill it, etc. The father looked at me in disbelief especially because I told him his son should not be eating any more game. I gave him a prescription for an antihistamine and told him to return the next day—which obviously he was not about to do. In the chart I wrote, "father not very bright—did not seem to understand what I told him"(!!). It was only on the ship taking me back to Europe that I realized that cantaloupe was a fruit because it was being served to us as a dessert!

Baroness Ghislaine D. Godenne, MD
Baltimore, MD

∅

Eric, a 5-year-old boy, came into our office with a temperature and an earache. I told Eric, "Don't worry, Dr Russo will fix you and you will be fine."

Eric's eyes became as big as saucers, and he began to cry. I was puzzled and looked at the mother, who smiled at me and said, "We just had our dog fixed."

Voja Russo, MD
Great Falls, VA

∅

The setting: A small exam room in a pediatric walk-in clinic at a Boston hospital
The year: 1975
The cast: An extended family from Puerto Rico whose 8-year-old child presented with a minor medical complaint; plus me, a pediatric chief resident with limited foreign language skills

After some preliminary introductions, I began a review of systems by asking the child if she had a headache.

"Tiene dolor en su cabeza?"

"No," she replied; she did not have a headache.

"Tiene dolor en sus ojos?"

"No," there was no eye pain.

"Tiene dolor en sus orejas?"

"No," she did not have an earache.

"Tiene dolor en su boca?"

"No," her mouth did not hurt.

"Tiene dolor en su bisabuelo?"

And with this, the entire room erupted in laughter. I grew red in the face and became even more embarrassed when I learned that the correct word for throat was *garganta,* whereas *bisabuelo* meant "great-grandfather."

Which synapses had crossed to cause this international faux pas I will never know, but I learned that this family (and many others since then) appreciated my attempt to communicate with them in their native language.

PS: Earlier this year, I took an intensive 4-day course in medical Spanish that should help me in future interviews—if I get a better grip on my vocabulary.

Carl S. Ingber, MD
Pebble Beach, CA

✆

I began my practice in Ft Yukon, Alaska, 8 miles north of the Arctic Circle, in a small Episcopal hospital. This is the land of permafrost…the ground stays frozen for hundreds of feet down, even though in the brief and intense summer it may be 90 degrees. For generations the Indians had been digging shafts in the permafrost by building a fire, thawing a few inches, digging, building another fire, etc. I was fascinated by these ice holes. So ingenious. They would have a year-round refrigerator to keep berries in, etc. Just climb down the ladder into a 10-foot deep ice pit in the ground. One day the native who was in charge of maintenance said, "Doc, me and the boys have been talking. What with your southern accent, and all, we think you need to stop talking about ice holes. We Indians are misunderstanding you."

S. Donald Palmer, MD
Sylacauga, AL

∅

A young man named Brian was in for his last visit with me; he had reached the age to leave my pediatric practice. Having a good rapport with teenagers, he told me a joke and I told him one.

As he was leaving, I said, "Brian, we found snew in your blood."

He replied, "What is snew?"

I said, "What's new with you?"

We both laughed, shook hands, and he left.

Later, my receptionist received a telephone call from the mother. She wanted to know what his lab results were and what "snew" was. Seems he didn't get the joke after all.

Claude A. Frazier, MD
Asheville, NC

∅

I was working as a nursing instructor in St Louis, MO, in 1979 and I was in the pediatric unit of a local hospital. One of the patients we were taking care of was a 3-year-old female with osteomyelitis (infection of the bones) who had already been in the hospital for 2 weeks. The total length of hospitalization was to be 6 to 8 weeks for IV antibiotics. At the time, central lines were not done, so she had to have numerous sticks—not only for IVs, but also for daily labs.

To help her express her feelings, we decided to do some play therapy. We gave her syringes and a tourniquet and left her alone with her "equipment" and her Kermit the Frog doll as her "patient." As we watched from the door, she placed the tourniquet around the frog's arm and proceeded to take one of the syringes and jab it into the bend of the arm. She then said, "Whoops, I missed! I'll have to stick you again!"

Mary Williamson, RN
Falls Church, VA

℘

I know electrocardiograms. I've spent my life doing ECGs. No one does a better ECG than I, getting just what is needed every time. I have made all the mistakes it is possible to make—or so I thought.

It wasn't very long ago that I was doing an ECG on a little 5-year-old boy. He was healthy, chipper, pink, and generally fine, but on his ECG, he was dead—nothing but a straight line. I checked everything, made sure all the leads were on properly, and was at a loss. After several minutes, in the disgusted tone of voice that only a 5-year-old dealing with stupid adults uses, he said "Doctor. Maybe if you plugged the wires you have attached to me into the machine it would work better." Ahhh! The humiliation.

Less than a week went by and I was in the same scenario but, fortunately, with a different boy. I learn from experience, so I checked and the cable was plugged into the machine. Another few minutes, and I heard exactly the same tone of voice as this boy said to me, "Doctor, maybe it would work better if you tried to do it on the machine you have me hooked up to."

New office rule: no more than one ECG machine in a room.

Chloe G. Alexson, MD
Rochester, NY

Chapter 10

From the Mouths of Babes

A 3-year-old was being seen for the first time. While taking the history, I asked him where he got the flaming red hair that was hanging down into his face. He promptly answered, "The mailman." His mother turned the same color as her son's hair and wanted to crawl under the exam table. We laughed about this story for many years.

Neal McNabb, MD
Honeoye Falls, NY

✆

A 5-year-old boy came in with his mother for some medical problem. At the end of the visit, the little boy asked, "When is the doctor coming in?"

The mother replied, "Dr Oswald *is* a doctor."

To which the boy quickly and firmly said, "No, she is not the doctor."

I told him, "Yes, I am the doctor."

He looked at me in a funny way and said, "But you are a girl. Doctors are boys."

The mother looked at me, embarrassed, and proceeded to explain to the little guy.

Leticia Oswald, MD
McLean, VA

✆

I was talking to a 12-year-old boy about puberty, explaining that in puberty his body would change from that of a child to that of a man. I asked him if he could think of something that happened to a boy's body when he grew up. He thought about it for a while, and then looking over at his father, inspiration struck him. His eyes lit up as he realized he knew the answer, and proudly replied, "You get fatter!"

Jon Matthew Farber, MD
Alexandria, VA

✆

Mrs Rosenfeld, a rabbi's wife, was a most proper lady. She had let me know in so many ways how much she appreciated my care of her only child, 5-year-old Rebecca.

From the day I first met Mrs Rosenfeld, and on every occasion thereafter, she would tell me about her concern for the lack of civility and manners in our children. She had raised Rebecca to be sensitive to others' feelings. She taught her to often use the 2 magic phrases: please and thank you. Rebecca was taken to events such as the opera and exposed to adult conversation as much as possible.

Rebecca came in for her pre-kindergarten examination, and her mother handed me a box of home-baked treats and an accompanying card that was most flattering. During my examination of Rebecca, Mrs Rosenfeld continued to expand on the subject of children's manners and informed me that Rebecca was limited to friends who were respectful of their elders and so on.

At the completion of my examination and on their departure, Mrs Rosenfeld turned to Rebecca and said, "Now what are you going to say to nice Dr Christu?" To which she responded, "You have a big nose, Dr Christu."

Chris N. Christu, MD
Minneapolis, MN

After I set up shop in a new practice, one of my first moves was to arrange a section with some treats in the left lower drawer of my desk. These treats included assorted cookies, candies, and carefully selected dime-store toys.

My first experiment with this plan was directed to a 6-year-old boy whom I had seen for an acute sore throat. After the visit I pulled out my left lower drawer and invited him to take whatever he liked. He began to fill up all of his available pockets with virtually my entire inventory. His mother was aghast and told him to put back everything but one item.

He replied, "But Dr Mac said I could take whatever I liked and I like it all!" (As a believer in both written and verbal contracts, I sided with the boy this time—but that never happened again!)

Campbell W. McMillan, MD
Chapel Hill, NC

✍

A young teenager came to see me for the first time. He was nicely dressed and accompanied by his fastidious and very concerned mother.

We needed to introduce a new medication and were discussing the possibility of a drug rash when she asked me to take a closer look at the rash he had on his arms and legs. She thought it was related to his current medicine.

I first asked whether it was itchy—no.

Then how long had it been there—weeks.

I took a closer look—patchy, irregular, somewhat pigmented appearing, certainly not red or irritated looking skin.

I knew exactly what it was and grabbed an alcohol swab and proceeded to wipe the rash away.

I'm sure this young man received a major lesson on bathing and using a washcloth. And perhaps his mom learned a good lesson too—think of the common things, not the rare and dangerous ones.

Patti Vining, MD
Baltimore, MD

℘

I was examining a 3-year-old with seasonal allergies. While looking in his nose, he said, "Doctor, do you know what's in there?"

I said, "What?"

"Boogies!" he replied with a smile.

"Well, I don't see any," I said with a chuckle.

"That's because I ate them all!" he exclaimed.

With this, his mother buried her face in her hands while turning bright red.

Lara Q. Barringer, MD
Owings Mills, MD

℘

My colleague was evaluating a 3-year-old girl with cervical adenitis and associated torticollis (pain in the neck). She was grunting, and the doctor was trying to figure out why. Was she in pain? When asked, the little girl answered, "I grunt when I am frustrated, and Mommy does it too."

Name withheld at sender's request

℘

A 14-year-old boy had an office visit with my partner for a complaint of knee pain. After an extensive exam, nothing was found, including any pain. So my partner told the boy and his mother to come back in a week if the pain returned. Worried, as most mothers are, the patient and the mother returned to see me a couple of days later for a second opinion. After another complete exam, I asked the boy, "When does your knee hurt?"

He replied, "When I hit it with a hammer!" Needless to say, the mother practically fell through the floor.

Ira S. Rubin, MD
Naperville, IL

℘

I saw a 7-year-old for a complaint of cough for a week. The father stated during the visit that he had been coughing for a while too, and that he was taking something for it every night, but he could not remember the name of the medication. He then asked his son, "What is that stuff that I have been taking every night?" His son answered, "Beer."

Francisco Enriquez, MD
Milwaukee, WI

Chapter 11

The Irrepressible Logic of Children

Part II

I do magic for the children as part of my routine exam. One trick is to make a quarter disappear and then make it reappear from a child's ear. (I only perform this on children old enough to know not to put things in their ears.) One time, while still in my residency at a large inner-city hospital, I was holding the coin after making it reappear when the child grabbed it from my hand. "That is my coin," I explained expecting him to give it back. "That is *my ear*," explained the child. I could not disagree with him, and let him keep the coin.

Richard Weil, MD
Atlanta, GA

✆

A teenager came to see me with a 2-week history of pain that extended from his right thigh to his ankle. When I asked him where the pain began, he said, "North Carolina."

Howard J. Bennett, MD
Washington, DC

✆

One night, my nurse was out with her husband at a movie. She kept hearing all of these whispers 2 rows behind her. Finally, at the end of the movie, she heard "That's Ms Patsy, but that's *not* Dr Stephen" in a very concerned tone.

Stephen P. Combs, MD
Gray, TN

While visiting Germany, 4-year-old Rebecca was listening to a small portable radio, which her parents had taken along from the United States. After a while, she remarked with much admiration for the radio, "This is a very smart radio. In America it speaks English and here in Germany it knows German."

Claus Helbing, MD
Annandale, VA

℘

As pediatricians and mothers we often deal with moral issues, and we look forward to those "teachable moments" to instill our wisdom in our children. When my daughter was about 5 years old, I began seeing a premature infant with his 14-year-old mother in my practice. My numerous conversations with this young mom at work and at home led to my daughter asking about her. I had the perfect opportunity to discuss the difficulties of being a teenager with a baby, and thus the importance of finishing school and being married before having a child.

Not long after this, we visited a young cousin of mine in Florida. She was a teacher and was engaged to be married a few months later. My daughter wanted to know if she had any children, and of course I again took the opportunity to reinforce our previous teachable moment. "No," I said, "she is not married yet."

That summer we went to my cousin's wedding up in New York, and my daughter sat through the entire ceremony without a peep. She seemed fascinated by the event and was so happy to see her cousin again. After the traditional stomping of the glass and "the kiss," the bride and groom came down the aisle right past my daughter. She immediately turned to me and said, "Mom, is she going to the hospital now to have her baby?"

I guess she was listening.

Susan Kohn, MD
Fairfax, VA

℘

When I do well-child checkups I like to ask my patients what they'd like to be when they grow up. One 3-year-old's answer: "Four."

Gail S. Hertz, MD
York, PA

℘

As a young pediatrician in the late 1930s, and having 2 small children of my own, I found Dr Gesell's books on child growth and development to be indispensable, both in my practice and at home.

One Sunday at family dinner, my 4-year-old son, Stevie, in his high chair next to Grandma, was happily wolfing creamed chicken and peas, one foot rhythmically kicking against the leg of the dining table. Grandma gently asked him to stop, it bothered the grown-ups. The respite was short and the thumping resumed. After a second reminder proved ineffective, Grandma's patience thinned. Scowling, she started to utter a stronger rebuke when Stevie interrupted.

"Why don't you look in the Gesell book and see if I'm not *supposed* to be doing this when I am 4 years old?"

Surprised, we consulted Gesell. Stevie was right!! We moved his high chair back from the table—until he passed through that developmental stage.

Elinor Fosdick Downs, MD
Boston, MA

✆

Development tests are important parts of any physical exam in children. She seemed very bright, knew her colors, and could count to 20, which is pretty good for a 4-year-old. She identified animals, drew a person, and could print her name. I was impressed. When I asked if she could hop on 1 foot, she acted stumped, but only for a second. She scratched her head, then smiled, and jumped heavily onto my left foot. As I limped into the next exam room, I wondered which psychologist thought up that test item.

Carl A. Salsbury, MD
Falls Church, VA

✆

A 5-year-old who had gone to summer camp was asked to tell her mother to give her a bottle of water to drink during the next session. Apparently the teacher had said something about how good it is to be hydrated, and the

5-year-old commented to her mother, "it is better to be hydrated than 'lowdrated,' I guess."

Mary Ellen Avery, MD
Boston, MA

℘

A 6-year-old boy with tonsillitis and sore throat came in. Johnny was not so sick and wanted very much to go to the swimming pool.

His mother said, "Dr Evers, Johnny wants in the worst way to go swimming, but I told him he's sick and can't go."

I looked in the throat and, sure enough, his tonsils were coated with infection. It had to be strep. I said, "Johnny, you're sick with a bad throat infection. I'm sorry, but you must stay home and be treated."

"But Doctor, I want to go to the swimming pool."

"Johnny, you have a lot of bugs in your throat and other boys and girls will get infected."

Looking at me with pleading blue eyes and a sorrowful half smile, he replied, "But I'll keep my mouth shut!"

Joseph C. Evers, MD
McLean, VA

My 5-year-old patient was a beautiful blue-eyed little girl. While my nurse was preparing her for the physical, she asked, "Where did you get your beautiful eyes?"

The girl replied in a matter-of-fact tone, "I've had them since birth."

Name withheld at sender's request

✀

After taking care of a 4-year-old boy and prescribing his medication, the mother and the boy were walking out the door when he said to his mom, "Dr Schweisthal is not very smart, is he?"

His mother asked him, "Why do you say that?"

The boy replied, "Well, he said I had a middle ear infection and I only have two ears; one on this side and one on the other side. I don't have a middle ear!"

Paul Schweisthal, MD
Vienna, VA

Chapter 12

Shots and Needles!

I remember an encounter with a child who was to have blood drawn. As I prepared to insert the needle into his vein he (naturally) started to cry and immediately turned his head away from his arm and faced the wall because he didn't want to look at the needle. I was taking my time drawing blood while he went on crying. Then suddenly he said, "Doctor, please tell me when you take the needle out of my arm so I'll know when to stop crying!"

Raphael David, MD
New York, NY

℘

I was called from eating lunch in our meeting room at the back of the office to see a little boy named Bradley, who had just been brought in from the playground with the story that he had been bitten by a snake. I examined the site of the alleged bite and found nothing, certainly not the fang marks of a poisonous snake.

"What did this snake look like, Bradley?" I asked.

"Oh, it was very big, and long, and black. And it had big teeth!"

Knowing that there were no poisonous snakes around here, and seeing no punctures, I commented, "You know, Bradley, if you were bitten by a snake, we would have to give you a lot of shots to keep you from getting sick."

Immediately he blurted out, "It was a fly!"

Lawrence F. Nazarian, MD
Rochester, NY

When I came to work in our evening clinic, I heard there was a 9-year-old girl hiding under a chair in one of the exam rooms, afraid to come out. I entered the room and found Sara under a chair in a panic that she was to receive the first in a series of 3 hepatitis B shots. It seems she has always had an extreme fear of needles. Because I knew her well, I asked if she would come out of her fortress so we could talk. When I promised her we would only talk, she reluctantly came out for air. Any mention of the shot sent her back, huddled in her fetal position under the chair. We talked about fears and how strong they can be.

Sara finally started talking about how scared she felt. After 45 minutes, I was able to bring out the syringe with the needle so she could look at it. I then gradually brought the needle closer to her arm, held it 1 inch from her arm for 10 minutes until she said, "Go!" and I gave her the shot. Sara looked at me and asked, "Is that all there is?"

One month later she showed up at my office and said only I could give her the shot. This time it only took 5 minutes!

Mark J. Mendelsohn, MD
Charlottesville, VA

✆

I had an 11-year-old female patient who was waiting to get her blood drawn for a blood test. She was quite nervous and upset and was giving the lab technician a lot of excuses about why they shouldn't poke her with a needle.

Finally, in tears, she said, "Can't you just wait until I fall down and scrape my knee and get the blood that way?"

Diana Mahar, MD
Oakland, CA

✆

I recently cared for a new family in our practice that had just adopted a 1-year-old girl from China. When I inquired as to any immunizations the child had received in the orphanage in China, the parents presented me with an immunization record written in Chinese. I suggested that they take the schedule to the local Chinese restaurant to have it translated. I received a copy of the translation, which described the immunizations for "the one hundred day cough," the "white throat," and "the shot for when cut with a dirty knife"—a literal but accurate translation.

Russell S. Asnes, MD
Tenafly, NJ

✆

In the clinic you could hear this woman's voice in every examining room, "I want a penicillin shot!"

I stepped outside into the corridor to find my colleague speaking to a mother, trying to assure her that her child had a simple cold and needed no antibiotics.

She persisted, "I want a penicillin shot!"

Again, he patiently explained—but the mother was not to be put off. "I want a penicillin shot!" After a couple more attempts, my colleague gave up, turned on his heels and spoke to the nurse who had been amusedly witnessing the interchange. Pointing to the woman's gluteus, he said, "Nurse, give this woman a penicillin injection!"

The mother, somewhat pale now, quietly retreated.

Angel Colon, MD
Bonita Springs, FL

✒

Lindsay was a 4-year-old girl scheduled for a shot visit. She was in the waiting room crying repeatedly, "I'm not sick, I'm not sick!" for a full 5 minutes. When Lindsay was in the exam room, she looked up with red-rimmed, tear-filled eyes and said to the nurse, "I might cry."

The nurse replied, "It's OK to cry. I'll be quick."

Right after the shot, Lindsay said her treat was to go to the car wash and then gave my nurse a big hug and a kiss.

Name withheld at sender's request

Chapter 13

Potty Humor

Many years ago I was teaching a class at a university medical school designed to convince first-year students about the pleasantness of the pediatrician's practice. After some discussion, an infant was brought in for me to examine and interact (play) with. The infant was good-natured, smiling, cute, and cuddly and was propped in my arm, with diaper at my wrist—the perfect patient. Naturally, and quite without warning, the infant looked up at me, smiled angelically, and proceeded to pass a very large, very watery, foul-smelling stool, which filled the diaper and ran onto my sleeve and hand. I don't think that any of those students selected a career in pediatrics.

Joe Zanga, MD
Maywood, IL

A 12-year-old named John was being helped by an inexperienced person because we had a nurse out sick. The assistant was nervous and tried to make John feel comfortable. She invited him to sit; there was a stool behind him. She said, "John, sit up there and have a stool."

He frowned and nervously said, "OUT HERE in front of everybody?"

She had meant to say, "Sit on the stool."

Claude A. Frazier, MD
Asheville, NC

A worried father called the on-call physician at 11:00 pm to report that his sleeping 3-year-old had not stooled in 3 days. He was reassured and advised to purchase some milk of magnesia. He called back at 6:00 am to again report that his sleeping child had still not stooled!

Jim Baugh, MD
Fairfax, VA

☙

One mother called me to relate that her 4-year-old boy smeared some dog droppings on his face and she wanted to know what disease that could cause.

I told her the child could not get rabies from that end of the dog. She wanted more information, about worms, etc. Finally I asked her if the dog was pedigreed. When she replied, "Yes," I told her that she had nothing to worry about. She broke into a laugh and it ended, or seemed to end, her concern.

A sense of humor is helpful in practice, and in life.

Milton Markowitz, MD
West Hartford, CT

My son was precocious in language, if not in motor skills, and we played to his strengths by using correct anatomic terms for various body parts. I knew we had gone too far when he was 3 years old and still working on wiping himself on the toilet and I heard from the bathroom, "Dad, come here! I got poop on my *spectacles!*"

Stephen Sulkes, MD
Rochester, NY

℘

Paul's mother was very concerned about the 18-month-old's green stools until I explained that they were due to the child's Irish heritage. She seemed satisfied with that explanation, and because the child had not lost any weight and was perfectly happy, I decided to leave it at that.

Carl A. Salsbury, MD
Falls Church, VA

Chapter 14

Parent Parade
Part II

A few years ago I walked into a patient room to check a baby for a 2-month well check. After chatting with the mother and reviewing the chart, I prepared to examine the child. Noting some noisy breathing and nasal congestion, I reached for the bulb and suctioned out the mouth and nose. The mother asked, "Where can I buy those things?"

I motioned to the bulb and said, "Any drug store. Did you lose the one you got at the hospital when she was born?"

"No, but *that* one is full now; I need another."

Mark Pashayan, MD
Winston-Salem, NC

✆

When told that her child had pneumonia, the mother of a 3-year-old asked, "Doctor, does she have the pneumonia just in the lungs or all over?"

George S. Palmer, MD
Tallahassee, FL

✆

Returning 2 weeks after treatment for an ear infection, the 2-year-old still had an infected ear. That's not overly unusual, but the mother was complaining that I had ordered much too much medication. My usual custom is to order the exact amount needed and no more, so I asked how often she had given the 3-times-a-day amoxicillin. She insisted that she had given the medicine as directed, but felt that I had overestimated the size of her child's ear canal as it would barely hold a half a teaspoon of the medication.

Carl A. Salsbury, MD
Falls Church, VA

✍

One Christmas Eve at about 2:00 am, I received a phone call. The mother explained that her infant had a diaper rash and she was worried. I asked how long the rash had been there. She stated that the infant had the rash about a month.

Ira S. Rubin, MD
Naperville, IL

✍

A panic-stricken parent called our office from Australia because her toddler had partially closed the car door on her hand, and her child was crying a lot. She was instructed to open the car door! There was no laceration or bone injury, fortunately, as determined by a local physician.

Jim Baugh, MD
Fairfax, VA

✍

Once upon a time, I provided a telephone hour. The line for most callers was always busy, and it didn't do much to facilitate accessibility for the patient. This was a long time ago. One morning, toward the end of the hour, the front doorbell rang. It was a Western Union messenger. The message from Mrs Smith: "Please call me before you leave the house."

Henry M. Seidel, MD
Baltimore, MD

℘

It was New Year's Eve, 1952. Few doctors were around. My answering service caught me as I was making 1 of the 25 house calls I made that night. "Doctor, there's a very sick 3-month-old. Their doctor is away and we can't find anyone for the family." I agreed to go. It was snowing heavily when I arrived at about 11:00 pm. A noisy, happy New Year's Eve party was in full swing. The child had pneumonia and was also quite croupy. I gave a shot of penicillin, wrote a prescription, and gave instructions for the baby's overnight care.

I had always used ipecac syrup (which is no longer recommended) in my treatment of croup. When told that the family had none in the house, I asked for a small container so that I could leave them some from the bottle that I always carried in my bag. The mother gave me a jigger glass, which I filled. She placed this on top of her refrigerator.

The next morning, New Year's Day, as instructed, the mother called me to report that the baby was much better. As we completed our conversation, the mother asked if I could call the pharmacy to order more ipecac. I quickly asked what had happened to the almost 2 ounces I had left them. Mom said, "The baby is much better, but my father-in-law is very bad. He thought someone had left their drink on the refrigerator, wanted to play a joke, and thus drank all of the ipecac in one gulp. He's been vomiting constantly ever since." She laughed a little. I called the pharmacy. Grandpa survived.

David Annunziato, MD
East Meadow, NY

℘

I had been taking care of a family from the Middle East. They returned to their home country for a visit, and I received an emergency call soon after they left. The call was from Qatar. The mother told me her 2-year-old son had a temperature of 102 degrees and asked what she should do. I fortunately knew a pediatrician in Qatar and suggested she take the child in to be seen by him. This was my *longest* long-distance telephone consultation.

James E. Strain, MD
Denver, CO

℘

Our son, Steve, was not particularly fastidious about keeping his room in order. I had asked a family to discuss with me some of their problems one evening. I chose to ask them to come to our home rather than my office. A real point of contention was the neglect the 14-year-old young man in that family manifested in the care of his room and his personal toilet. "No problem," said I. I invited them upstairs to visit our son's room (he was out at a school function). It was in absolutely splendid order! My wife had been up there barely a half an hour before to straighten things out!

Henry M. Seidel, MD
Baltimore, MD

℘

Here is a brief snippet taken from a medical history:
    Pediatrician: "What is your little boy's problem?"
    Patient's mother: "Pain in the textiles." (She meant *testicles.*)

Grange S. Coffin, MD
Berkeley, CA

℘

I just had completed a well-child visit on a 5-year-old and was about to leave the room when the real reason for the visit became apparent. When my hand was on the doorknob, she said, "My husband just left me. Do you think it is going to affect the children?" Because I was already 30 minutes behind in my scheduled appointments, I asked if she would mind coming in again to talk about it because this could be a problem that could conceivably affect her children. She agreed.

In an effort to include all of the essentials of a well-child visit, we sometimes fail to pick up on what is really important to the child and the family.

James E. Strain, MD
Denver, CO

Chapter 15

The Joys of Pediatrics

It was a long and tiring day at the hospital clinic. I was an intern in a hot exam room with my last patient and his siblings, all under the age of 5. Tongue depressors, alcohol pads, and paper towels were strewn about, all over the floor. A devilish 4-year-old boy was bouncing up and down on the exam table. As I finished the exam, the youngster begged for—and then grabbed for—my stethoscope. I usually do not relinquish, but this time, fatigue made me cave in to his request. When I returned to see them off, he smiled and said, "Thank you for giving me my heart."

That is why I chose the field of pediatrics.

Laura Voigt, MD
Arlington, VA

℘

One day as I was examining a child, I was at the point where I had a nasal speculum in his nose.

He said, "Eew, that's nasty!" And then he said, "Are you guys real doctors?"

I said, "Yes."

And he said, "You mean you guys go to medical school and all that hospital stuff after that?"

After I assured him we did, he then said, "Why do you have to go to school so long just to look at boogers!"

Gary S. Flom, MD
Stockbridge, GA

A little boy patient admitted for pneumonia in the medical side of a pediatric ward where I worked in 1953 asked a patient in the surgical side the difference between "medical" and "surgical" patients. The answer he got was: "a medical patient comes to the hospital sick and leaves well, a surgical patient comes in well and goes out sick."

Baroness Ghislaine D. Godenne, MD
Baltimore, MD

℘

"Where did you get all that red hair, Mike?" I asked a new patient hoping to distract him from the discussion of "shots." "I've never seen so much hair on a young boy's head."

"Well, I was born with it!" he said, emphatically, "Where is your hair?" pointing to my very bald scalp.

I suddenly made a quick motion to feel the top of my head, simultaneously registering feigned shock on my face, while I quickly walked over to the square wall mirror over the small washbasin, and exclaimed, "Oh my goodness! What happened to my hair?" I slowly turned to face Mike as I continued, feigning even greater shock than before, "It was there this morning when I came to the office and parked my car in the parking lot."

I noticed that Mike had suddenly become entranced.

"Do you think I might have lost it out in the parking lot, Mike?" I asked, as I continued to feel my scalp and began to return to the examining table.

By now I had picked up the instruments and had lain them down beside Mike. He didn't even notice my doing that, because his gaze was fixed on my shiny dome.

I knew I had his complete trust when he answered, "Well, maybe you can find it sometime."

I had absolutely no difficulty in examining Mike thereafter. In fact, he was most cooperative. After he'd dressed, he even gave me an affectionate hug.

I then proceeded to examine other patients, and had essentially put the conversation with Mike out of my mind entirely.

About an hour later, the nurse accosted me in the hall saying that Mike's mother was back in the waiting room wanting to speak with me.

"Doctor," she said, "I just had to come back to tell you what Mike has been doing since we left the office."

"Oh, I hope everything's all right. He didn't hurt himself, did he?"

"Oh, no! Not at all. Nothing like that," she said emphatically, breaking out into a full and pleasing smile. "You really made a wonderful impression on Mike, because the minute he walked out of your office, we went directly out the front door and he announced we had to look for your 'lost hair' in the parking lot! We've been looking for your hair in every nook and cranny of that lot for this entire time! He's convinced it's out there and he won't go home until we find it!"

Her next question was asked with an imploring tone, as she tilted her head slightly forward and downward, almost embarrassingly, "Would you please go out there and tell Mike the truth about your hair? He and his sister refuse to go home until they find it."

I went out through the rear entrance to the office so my other patients would not see me leave. Mike's mom and I arrived on the scene as Mike was looking under a pickup truck.

"Mike," I said to him as I raised him from the crouching position he had assumed to look under that truck, "Dr Davoli was only kidding about his hair. I was just trying to get you relaxed, so you wouldn't be scared of the doctor today."

Mike looked up at me, puzzled; I feared I might have just destroyed the rapport I'd recently enjoyed with him. However, after a few brief moments, he broke out into a big smile, and said, "Oh, you really wanted to fool me, Dr Davoli?"

"Of course, Mike. Is that OK?" I asked, hopefully.

"Sure," he responded quickly, and in almost the same breath, noticing his mom behind me, he said, enthusiastically, "Mom, did you know that Dr Davoli tried to fool me about his hair?"

Ah, another triumph, I said to myself, as I returned to my office to see the remaining patients.

I smiled throughout the rest of that day.

Enrico Davoli, MD
McLean, VA

(Reprinted in an edited form courtesy of Dr Davoli from his upcoming book House Calls and Other Nostalgia.*)*

✇

The following took place after I had been in practice quite a number of years. I walked into an examining room to find 2 women and an infant. The mother, a teenager, was cradling the baby in her arms and said,

"Oh, Dr Herndon, I wanted you to see my baby because you took care of me when I was little." I started to smile, when the second lady, her mother, said, "Yes, and you took care of me, too." Sometimes there can be almost too much of a good thing!!

Robert Herndon, MD
Chickasha, OK

✆

I'm sure many pediatricians have had this experience. It's happened to me more than once. A mother called at 3:00 am and began the conversation with "I hope I'm not disturbing you."

James E. Strain, MD
Denver, CO

✆

The absolute trust that children can develop in you as a physician is most humbling. There is no other profession that allows the same degree of enmeshment over such a long period as the practice of pediatrics.

When the letter announcing my impending retirement arrived in one household, the 10-year-old said to his mother, "You mean I can never go to the doctor again if I get sick?"

Beverley J. Bayes, MD
McLean, VA

One day, years ago, in our office of 5 pediatricians, our patients seemed louder and unhappier with being there than usual and, indeed, it was bedlam. A beautiful 3½-year-old girl, when she got up on the examining table, leaned over to me and in a reassuring manner said, "Doctor, I am not going to get mad at you!"

John F. Shriner, MD
Montrose, AL

✂

One blustery December day, I found a particularly terrified 3-year-old boy quivering on my examining table. A veritable mountain of winter clothing was piled beside him. His mother had succeeded in divesting him of everything except his underpants. These he gripped with 10 white knuckles, defying anyone in the world to take them down. But somehow, down they must come, because the purpose of the visit was to see if he had a hernia in his groin. His mother sat in the chair beside him looking up at me with a look of despair which seemed to say, "Doctor, I've done the very best I could, but he's *so* frightened."

Assuming complete control of the situation, I marched up to the little lad and said confidently, "Johnnie, I can tell you what you had for lunch."

Johnnie didn't utter a sound, but the defiant look on his face clearly said, "No, you can't."

Rubbing his tummy gently in a neutral area away from the disputed underpants, I announced after a grave pause, "Aha! PB and J."

The response to this pronouncement was most satisfactory. Clearly, this little boy had met a genius. There was no point in fighting a man who could tell just by rubbing your stomach that you had recently ingested peanut butter and jelly. Down came the underpants without further protest, and the necessary examination was quickly concluded.

"Well," I said triumphantly, "you had better get dressed now, hadn't you?" I've seen some pretty fast pants-putter-on-ers in my day, but this kid broke all records. He went from no underpants to full winter garb, including snowsuit, galoshes, hat, scarf, and mittens, in less than 20 seconds—all by himself. His mother sat there dumbfounded.

"Oh Doctor," she gushed, "you were so wonderful!"

I was about to say, "It's nothing, Mother, all kids his age eat peanut butter and jelly," when she added, "but you forgot to mention the apple he had for lunch!"

Looking at him humbly in the eye, I admitted, "Johnnie, you sure did fool me, 'cause I didn't feel any apple at all in your tummy."

Without lowering his gaze from mine, Johnnie slowly produced an apple from the depths of his snowsuit pocket and whispered solemnly, "I didn't eat it yet."

Surely rewards must come to physicians who care for adults, but what can compare to moments like these that enchant the life of a children's surgeon?

Thomas S. Morse, MD
Richmond, MA

(Reprinted with permission of the author from his book,
A Gift of Courage.)

Children have given me so many wonderful treasures over the years. The gaily colored pictures of myself they are so proud of, the crumpled handful of buttercups or dandelions that caught their eye, the sticky lifesavers or my favorite gummy bears, the lovely handmade cards that shower sprinkles all over the desk when I open the envelope. I have loved them all. But most of all they have given me themselves—open, honest, reactive, inquisitive, frightened, loving. Their generosity of spirit is their greatest gift of all.

Beverley J. Bayes, MD
McLean, VA

❧

In the 1950s, when I was in practice in North Carolina, I walked into the hospital room of 5-year-old Rudy. He was standing at the foot of his crib and greeted me with, "Hello Dr Hall. Does your face hurt?"

Taken aback, I said, "No."

Rudy said, "Well, it's killing me!"

I liked being on a joking basis with my little friends.

Incidentally, Rudy's mother telephoned me last month. Just checking on me after all these many years!

Rowena S. Hall, MD
Bethesda, MD

Chapter 16

Siblings

I walked into an exam room and a very pleasant 3-year-old boy was sitting on the exam table with his 2-year-old brother next to him. The 3-year-old had a large book in his hands and was telling the story and turning the pages in the book to the delight of his younger brother.

I asked the 3-year-old if he could read. The immediate response was, "Of course I can read, I'm three!"

I was very impressed and asked him if he could read the whole book. He answered, "Of course I can read the whole book; I can read everything except the letters parts."

David Monroe, MD
Columbia, MD

✆

This story was related to me by my preceptor: A 6-year-old boy waited for his appointment with his mother and younger 4-year-old brother. Because he was so patient and had been waiting quite a while, one of the nurses gave the young boy a piece of hard candy. The doctor heard screams coming from the room. The young boy was choking on the candy. The doctor performed the Heimlich maneuver and, after a few tries, was able to dislodge the candy. It popped out of the young boy's mouth and onto the floor. A sense of relief filled the room. Everyone was relieved at how the situation had turned out—except the 4-year-old younger brother. You see, as soon as the candy hit the floor, the youngster sprinted over to the candy, snatched it up, and just as quickly placed it back in his brother's mouth. How dare the evil doctor take candy from his brother!

Todd Denton Gould, MD
Charlottesville, VA

✆

I was examining a newborn and narrowly missed being showered. As his mom was changing him, his older brother piped up, "Mommy says he's going to be a fireman when he grows up 'cause he likes hosing people down."

Gail S. Hertz, MD
York, PA

✆

An adorable 7-year-old came to the office with her mother and 8-year-old brother. The girl complained of severe pain in the right ear for several days. She had no history of ear infections and had been perfectly healthy, without any upper respiratory infections, fever, sore throat, or allergy symptoms in the previous few weeks.

As I began my examination, it was clear that this girl was particularly frightened about having her ears touched. She squirmed and cried with even the gentlest attempts to look into the ears and, as is usual in a case like this, the canals were packed full with hard, dry wax. Due to her apprehension, I was unable to use a curette to remove the wax, so I explained calmly that her ears would be flushed with warm water. The little girl went silent and turned pale. She insisted her brother remain closely by her side during the lavage procedure. (Mom remained quietly seated in the corner of the room, embarrassed by her daughter's behavior.)

After a few syringes full of water were instilled into the canal, the sound of a gentle "clink" in the catch basin signaled success. A cute little baby tooth was sitting in the middle of the basin of water. Now the story poured out from the previously quiet little girl.

It seems the sister and brother had been wrestling (against house rules), when her brother landed a successful body slam, and out popped the already loose tooth. Fearing maternal wrath, the siblings were too afraid to confess the truth, so they quickly stashed the evidence into the nearest available hiding place. Like any little sister, the girl protested that her elder brother "made her do it, or else we'd be in big trouble." He did concede that the idea of hiding the tooth in the ear was his, and "it was a good idea because no one found out until now." (Surprisingly, no one noticed the space in the girl's mouth!)

The tooth fairy made the appropriate visit to that family's house that night, and the girl and I chuckle about where her other baby teeth have turned up once they've fallen out.

Julie McAndrews, MD
Vienna, VA

One day, as I was examining a young infant in the presence of his mother and 4-year-old sister, I turned him onto his abdomen, whereby he proceeded to move all extremities as if in a crawling fashion.

I commented, jokingly, "Gosh! Look at him! I wonder if he will crawl away."

Big sister replied, "I hope not, 'cause we just got him!"

Doug McDowall, MD
Fairfax, VA

✆

A mother of one of my patients relayed this story to me a few years ago.

This family already had three boys aged 17, 21, and 23, and there occurred one of those "unexpected" pregnancies. The parents decided to tell all 3 of the kids at one time that they would be getting a little brother or sister in a few months. The youngest brother stared at them blankly and then spouted out, "Oh Mother, that is disgusting!" The little sister is now 8 and the boys all spoil her as much as possible.

Emanuel O. Doyne, MD
Cincinnati, OH

✆

Two brothers, aged 3 and 4 years, were sitting on an exam table. As I entered the room, one poked the other and said, "See I told you we get the short fat one!"

Their mother looked like she was going to faint, and I was unable to stop laughing.

Marvin Tabb, MD
Silver Spring, MD

✆

One of my small patients, a $2\frac{1}{2}$-year-old who had been born with a cleft lip and palate that still required speech therapy, called me "Ocher Bees." One day when his little brother was crying loudly with an earache, he walked over, patted the baby on the head and said, "Don't worry. Ocher Bees will fix it."

Beverley J. Bayes, MD
McLean, VA

✆

Two brothers, aged 2 and 4, were sitting in church. As the powerful organ started playing, the younger one was startled. When he collected himself he pushed his brother and asked, "What is this?"

The older brother looked at his younger brother and replied knowingly, "This is a huge radio."

Claus Helbing, MD
Annandale, VA

The 4-year-old boy had heard his pediatrician refer to his genital area as plumbing. "Let's check your plumbing," he would say on checkups.

So when the boy saw his mother changing his new baby sister's diaper, he cried in a panic, "What happened to her plumbing?"

Parichehr Farsad, MD
Rochester, NY

☙

I was examining an infant on the exam table. While I looked in the baby's ears, she cried heartily. The 3-year-old sibling came up in defense of the baby and kicked me in the shin!

All in a day's work!

Patricia Rappaport, MD
Alexandria, VA

Chapter 17

Training Days

A nurse once told me this story: Her husband was a surgical resident and had the usual terrible surgical hours, coming home exhausted every other night, and usually late. They had a 3-year-old daughter. One night her husband came home late and, sitting down before dinner, decided to have a martini. In their small apartment his wife (the nurse) was talking to him from the kitchen, around the corner from their living room. As she was chatting away she realized she was getting no response, so came around the corner to see what was going on. There he was, head back in the stuffed chair, sound asleep, his daughter playing quietly at his feet. She said, disgustedly, "Oh, he's gone off to sleep again!"

Their daughter, looking up from the floor, got up and, pushing his eyelid up and peering into his eye, said, "No, Mommy, he's not gone anywhere, he's right in there."

Will Cochran, MD
Boston, MA

Dr Lewis Barness has been one of the icons of pediatrics for almost a half century. He gained rather significant notoriety back in the 1960s (and beyond) for carrying a water pistol in his lab coat pocket. Medical students and especially residents were often on the receiving end of a volley of water on rounds if they did not know the answer to one of the "Chief's" questions. He later discovered that a 10-cc syringe provided greater distance, accuracy, and volume than the water pistol. More than once he was on the receiving end of the volley, usually from rotating interns on their last day on pediatric service. The Chief could receive as well as give.

Dr Barness frequently served as one of the "checkers" in well-child clinic. Students and interns were required to present their patients to the checker, who would review the history and physical examinations and the management plans, which almost always included immunizations. The Chief had received a pink, fluorescent replica of a syringe, probably from one of the drug companies. It was large enough to require 2 hands to carry. Naturally, he brought the toy with him to clinic. A medical student presented his patient to the Chief, including plans for immunizations, which he had already drawn up into a syringe. The Chief, after hearing the student's presentation, accompanied him into the examining room, fluorescent syringe in his arms. Unwittingly, the student had told the mother of the infant that he would be right back with the shots. The blur of the mother and infant running out of the room was memorable!

Walter W. Tunnessen, Jr, MD
Chapel Hill, NC

Once when I was a resident, I was entering an isolation ward in my white gown and puffy white paper hat. The little girl who I was to examine looked at me with wide eyes and asked, "Are you the baker?"

Ronald Schmidt, MD
Anniston, AL

(now retired to Newnan, GA)

A student took a family history of a patient with enuresis. He had asked the mother if anyone in the family had a history of enuresis. She seemed to recoil at the idea and denied it. In reviewing the case with the student I tried again, but asked whether anyone in the family wet the bed. The mother proceeded to list various close family members who had prolonged bed-wetting and then added that she, herself, had wet the bed up to 19 years of age. The student later agreed that it was best to use nonscientific terms when taking a medical history.

David Mosier, MD
Irvine, CA

When I was working in the outpatient clinic at a hospital, I had the habit of supplying some orange juice and graham crackers, which stayed near the counter where the records of patients-to-see were stacked and waiting. The crackers and juice were quick supplements to help us survive the long exhausting afternoons. One afternoon, I arrived at the clinic and was startled to see a very good resident feeding a little boy who was under treatment for presumed celiac disease (sensitivity to wheat and other grains). He was feeding orange juice and the whole-wheat crackers to a patient with celiac diarrhea! The resident was enjoying this and the patient was having the time of his life! Later I heard the boy did not have a setback and did continue to improve. So cheering up was good treatment.

Grange S. Coffin, MD
Berkeley, CA

On my first day of residency at a hospital in Cincinnati, blood was ordered on a 4-year-old boy with Lupus who was very cushingoid (some obesity of the abdomen and the face). Apparently many previous attempts had been unsuccessful, although I was unaware. With luck I found a vein and was successful. The young patient looked at me and said, "You done good, Doc!"

What a way to start a residency!

Jacqueline A. Noonan, MD
Lexington, KY

✍

The 2½-year-old was as endearing as any child we had taken care of as pediatric interns. He followed us on rounds, clung to our legs, and smiled easily and constantly. Nurses, residents, and students alike could not help but respond positively to the youngster. His acute medical problem was not a major one, but he clearly was microcephalic (had a small head), and this usually portends mental retardation.

A few days after admission, as the ward team gathered around the youngster's crib, our attending physician led a discussion on microcephaly and a review of developmental milestones.

"How do you account for the apparent discrepancy between this youngster's normal developmental milestones and his microcephaly?" commanded our attending.

One of our group responded immediately to this apparent paradox. "A small but powerful brain!" came the quick retort.

Walter W. Tunnessen, Jr, MD
Chapel Hill, NC

✆

While in medical school, an upperclassman was obtaining the family history from a patient's mother:

"Are your parents living?""

"No," the mother replied, "They passed away a few years ago."

"Oh, what did they die of?"

"Nothing serious," she replied.

Mohsen Ziai, MD
Falls Church, VA

✆

Although we are led to believe that we in the United States speak the same language as they do in the United Kingdom, don't believe it. As a medical student on rotation in Britain, I found misunderstandings to be daily occurrences. One day I volunteered to go and see a newly admitted patient.

"I think it is my turn. I will go and work up the patient this afternoon."

Dead silence followed by, "Don't you think you should just do your history and physical and not get her upset?"

Apparently in the UK, one does one's history and physical by "clerking" rather than "working up" a patient.

Peter D. Grundl, MD
Falls Church, VA

✆

Many years ago, I was a junior resident at a hospital in Washington, DC. It was 2:00 am and I was on duty in the emergency department. A nice grandmother brought her granddaughter to the hospital because of a fever. She told me, "Doctor, I think my granddaughter has pneumonia, I will pray for you if you admit her."

She further explained that a few years ago she took another child of her family to some other hospital for fever; the child was sent home where he died in the morning. After this conversation I did not even try to examine the patient and I immediately called my senior resident and told him the situation, and he, in turn, agreed with admission.

By the way, that child had pneumonia.

Iradj Mahdavi, MD
Rockville, MD

A student recounted his dialogue with the mother of a child:

"Any serious illnesses in your family?"

"Yes," she replied, "My sister developed *romantic* fever when she was 6 years old."

Mohsen Ziai, MD
Falls Church, VA

⌀

One can get into trouble, particularly when using language that might be just too professional for the audience. This is particularly a problem with medical students, unsure of their professional demeanor to begin with. Seems one such medical student was taking a history from a mother about her daughter.

"Now did the patient appreciate any abdominal pain last evening?"

"Of course she didn't appreciate it [you ninny], she was up crying all night long."

Peter D. Grundl, MD
Falls Church, VA

When I was a second-year medical student studying diligently for step 1 of the medical boards, I would stay up late at night. My daughter would watch me retire to the "dungeon" and begin the drudgery of studying facts about physiology and psychology, etc. When I was within a week of my test, I huffed out loud out of exasperation, "How will I ever learn *all* of this material?"

My 3-year-old daughter calmly replied, "Mommy, you can never know it all, just do your best!"

Madhu Henry, MD
Washington, DC

Chapter 18

Kids Say the Darndest Things
Part III

Diane was 3 years old when her parents, good friends of ours, brought her to see me for thumb sucking. I have had some success in this age group by making eye contact and directly speaking to the child about how she is a big girl now and won't need to suck her thumb anymore and how proud I am of her and how happy I'll be, and so on.

I did this with Diane. I saw her mom about 2 weeks later and asked her how Diane was doing. She said, "As we were leaving your office parking lot that very day I glanced back in the rearview mirror and saw Diane sucking her thumb. I said, 'Diane! What did Dr Byrd say to you about that?' Diane pulled her thumb out of her mouth with a loud sucking sound and replied, 'I don't care if he's happy or not!'"

Richard L. Byrd, MD
Sugar Land, TX

℘

On bedside rounds, we were discussing the problems with the electrolytes (sodium, potassium, chloride, and bicarbonate) in a 7-year-old boy.

After rounds, he asked me, "Dr Cohen, what's wrong with my electric lights?"

Solomon J. Cohen, MD
New York, NY

On a trip to an asthma camp in West Virginia, our family had a stopover in a motel with an outdoor swimming pool. After a hot day of driving, the children were anxious to get into the pool. Three-year-old Ina had to check it out as soon she got out of the car. She ran to the pool and returned with a sad face. "Daddy, Daddy," she proclaimed, "there are 'allergies' in the pool." She was very happy to hear that she could go into the pool. The "allergies" were algae, which were no health hazard.

Claus Helbing, MD
Annandale, VA

❡

Because of our work on asthma in the inner city of New York, I have been interviewed on both local and national TV. One of my younger patients, a 4-year-old boy, on seeing me on the television screen in his living room, turned to his mother and asked, "How did Dr Mellins climb into the box?"

Robert B. Mellins, MD
New York, NY

❡

A few weeks ago, I had a delightful time examining a 3-year-old boy in my office. Although frightened at first, the boy warmed up when I let him play with my finger puppets and some of the other toys in my office. When it came time to do the genital exam, I asked him to pull down his underpants so I could check his penis. He looked puzzled for a moment and then said, "But I don't have any peanuts."

Howard J. Bennett, MD
Washington, DC

☙

I was checking a little girl's ears. To distract her, I told her that she had a squirrel in the first ear (a universal ruse!). Then, the second ear:
"You've got a varmint in this ear, too." I said.
She replied, "Yeah, I know. I *varmited* yesterday!"

S. Donald Palmer, MD
Sylacauga, AL

☙

My sister and 4-year-old niece accompanied my mother to an orthopedic appointment. The doctor came into the room and soon began to review the x-rays and CT scan. After a few minutes of the orthopedist placing and replacing films on the view box, my niece looked at my mother and said, "Boy, he's good!"

Kelly Bruce Lobley, MD
Spring, TX

He was cute and small and had a great smile for me as I entered the examining room. "S-E-X," he spelled and smiled.

I looked up and said, "Yes, Chris."

"S-E-X," he spelled again.

I again asked, "What about it, Chris?"

He looked at me, a bit aggravated because of my stupidity, and said loudly, "S-E-X, I'm *six!*"

Carl A. Salsbury, MD
Falls Church, VA

✆

A 4-year-old girl was in for a routine office visit. As I entered the examining room she was in, I noticed she was giving what appeared to be bubble gum a real workout. To make her comfortable, I said, "That must be good gum. What kind is it?" She looked me right in the eye and said, "It is the kind you chew the smell out of." I supposed that to be peppermint.

Claude A. Frazier, MD
Asheville, NC

✆

I had the following experience with my son one day. We were staying at a hotel in downtown Chicago. In the gym room everybody was busy on the various machines. My 6-year-old son got on one of those stationary bikes and started pedaling. Pretty soon he saw the number "40" on the screen for the caloric consumption. He turned around with a big grin on his face and told me "Look Dad, I lost forty pounds!" I looked at him and burst into laughter and asked him "Where are you, I can't see you!" In this era of obsession with weight loss, how little ones get cues from adults about what life should be.

Amar Dave, MD
Ottawa, IL

✄

The magical thinking that is so characteristic of young children provided an amusing anecdote when Jake, who was not quite 3, developed a viral illness with a high fever.

Having gone through training in the era of formal attire, I always wore a dress or skirt and blouse, nylon stockings, and a white coat in the office. The stockings were often a great fascination to the toddlers because many of them had never seen their mothers or other caretakers in anything but slacks or jeans. They would often toddle over and run their hands down my legs to try to figure out just exactly what these strange things were.

I didn't realize, however, that any of them ascribed magical powers to the stockings until Jake got sick. He felt so terrible; he said to his mother, "Take me to Dr Bayes and Dr Bayes' stockings. I need to feel better."

Beverley J. Bayes, MD
McLean, VA

One morning a little boy slips into my office and shouts with his "croupy" voice, "Doctor, I have a horse in my mouth. Please remove it!" "Who told you so?" I inquired. "My mother said so as I spoke this morning, she heard me and said, 'You have a hoarse voice. Let us take you to the doctor.'"

John G. Bitar, MD
McLean, VA

⌀

A 5-year-old boy with neck pain came to see me. He was in such discomfort, I couldn't even touch him. So I asked him to squeeze my hands as hard as he could. And I told him, "Oh boy! You are really strong. Do you take karate?" "No," he said, "I take medicine."

Sunny Thomas, MD
Warren, PA

⌀

Recently, a 2-year-old who had a history of recurrent otitis media and had received an antibiotic injection for treatment was here for follow-up. My nurse went to get the little boy, who was watching *Bear in the Big Blue House*. When he saw my nurse, he looked up and said, "Oh gawd."

Stephen P. Combs, MD
Gray, TN

One summer afternoon, a 3-year-old boy came into our community health center with his mother for his mandatory preschool physical. It was his first visit to our health center, and he was completely silent during the examination, despite my efforts to involve him in conversation. Despite his silence, however, he was clearly observant and quite cooperative. His mother and I chatted easily about his health history and, after examining him and filling out his preschool form, I saw them to the door. I bent down to the little boy and looked him in the eye.

"See you later alligator!" I said, smiling, not expecting any reply and certainly not the conventional one about crocodiles. The little boy looked at me solemnly. Then he said his first words to me, revealing just how observant (and creative!) he really was—"See you later, fish."

Paula Brinkley, MD
Tamuning, Guam

❦

Justin, a 6-year-old asthmatic, had come in after a few days of labored breathing. Reviewing his record I noted that he'd been prescribed a nebulizer for home use. I asked his mom if he'd been using the machine at home. Without skipping a beat Justin answered for himself, "Oh yes, I've used my SUV every day."

Joseph J. Wells, MD
Phoenix, AZ

A 6-year-old girl named Sandi came into our office with abdominal pains, diarrhea, a temperature, and vomiting. After the child was examined, I gave instructions to the patient's mother about diet and hydration, and told the child not to give those "presents" to her family. Sandi turned around and said, "Oh, don't worry, Dr Russo. Christmas is over and I already gave them my presents!"

Voja Russo, MD
Great Falls, VA

✄

A 4-year-old boy came to the receptionist window with his mother. The receptionist asked the mother which of the doctors she wanted to see. The mom had no strong feelings about which she would see but the little boy said, "I want to see the doctor who lets me cry." I have always felt the cry of a child is him telling us his feelings, and if they cooperate and pretty much do what we want, then I don't mind if they cry and express their feelings.

Paul Schweisthal, MD
Vienna, VA

✄

Five-year-old Alice looked solemn and a bit tentative as she entered my office. Her mother explained that Alice had a sore throat and hadn't wanted to eat or drink for a few days.

Alice didn't seem sick. She didn't say a word, she just watched. I lifted her onto the edge of the examining table and put a wooden tongue depressor to her lips. She bit down on it.

"No, honey...like this," and leaning down toward her I opened my mouth wide. She stared straight into my gaping mouth, paused a moment, then slowly opened hers.

Later, as her mother led her from the office, Alice looked timidly up at me. Breaking her silence for the first time, she asked seriously, "How come all your gold teeth are in the back instead of the front, where people can see them?"

Elinor Fosdick Downs, MD
Boston, MA

On one occasion a youngster came in with the chief complaint of bloody urine, and when asked his name, he replied, "Rusty Sprinkler."

Mary Ellen Avery, MD
Boston, MA

One day I was sitting at my computer during lunch trying out a dinosaur CD-ROM game I had bought for the office to entertain my patients as they waited for me. In walked little Sarah and asked if she could try it. "Sure," I said, and she hopped onto my lap. After a short while it was obvious that I was in the presence of a dinosaur expert. As she answered every question right and I answered every one wrong, she turned and said, "Doctor, you need a lot of work!"

Ed Lewin, MD
New York, NY

Chapter 19

Heartwarming Tales
Part II

In mid-December, a 10-year-old boy (whom I shall call Billy) was admitted for treatment of acute lymphoblastic leukemia on our pediatric hematology/oncology service. His disease had very unfavorable characteristics, and he died in our intensive care unit about 5 days before Christmas.

He had lived with foster parents virtually all of his life. They had been unable to have children of their own and took him as an infant. Then, 6 years later, the parents were overjoyed to add their own daughter (whom I shall call Sarah) to the family unit. Thereafter, Sarah bonded to Billy so thoroughly that the parents decided to follow through on their own long-standing love for Billy and their growing urge to adopt him. His adoption had been completed for about a year before he developed leukemia. At the time of his death Sarah was a little over 4 years old.

When the parents were summoned to inform them of Billy's death, Sarah insisted on being with them. After the conference, as customary, the parents were offered the opportunity of seeing Billy in his room. They chose to do so but, quite contrary to usual custom, Sarah insisted on going with them. With absolutely no understanding of what was in Sarah's mind and after a brief open exchange among us, we all went to Billy's bed. The intensive care unit resident, nurse, and I stood aside while the parents embraced Billy and grieved very appropriately. Sarah stood patiently at the foot of Billy's bed and did not shed a tear. After her parents finally reached a mutually perceived end point and pulled away from the bedside, Sarah took their place. She reached into her coat pocket, produced a small brown teddy bear, and placed it carefully in Billy's right hand. Then, still without a tear, she took her mother's hand and was ready to leave.

Campbell W. McMillan, MD
Chapel Hill, NC

℘

I was sitting on a bed with a patient who was scheduled for brain surgery. We both dangled our legs over the bed and she stared downward as I told her about the surgery, the expected results, the likelihood she was scared—the usual, if you will. I asked if she wanted to talk about anything that may be troubling her. I was prepared for the usual questions about death, disability, pain, and disfigurement. She paused for a while, continuing to stare downward, and then turned to me and said, "You know, Dr Adelman, you have the smallest feet."

Ray Adelman, MD
Phoenix, AZ

℘

During my hematology/oncology rotation at a hospital in Memphis, I cared for a young boy who had undergone surgery for a brain tumor. He was unable to swallow any foods and received his nutrition via tube and/or intravenously. One day I asked him if there was anything I could do to help him, and he said he would like a "loaded" baked potato with everything on it: sour cream, bacon, cheese, etc. He said that he knew he couldn't swallow it, let alone eat it, but he wanted to TASTE it, to FEEL it in his mouth. Needless to say, we got him his loaded baked potato!

Andrea Weaver, MD
Herndon, VA

✺

Many years ago, I had joined a hospital staff in Boston as a new teaching and research fellow. Because I was thousands of miles from home with no family nearby and no plans for the holidays, I felt very bleak. As I walked about the wards on rounds, facing the sickest children, I felt a certain compassionate empathy with them because we were all removed from home on this most family-centered of holidays. The play and recreation director came up to me and asked, "Do you have any plans for Christmas Eve tonight?" "No," I replied. "Then you can be our Santa!" she exclaimed. "The regular Santa is ill and can't be here." As a tall, skinny pediatrician not noted for any levity, I hesitated. "We have the suit all ready with the right padding and presents to pass out. You will be fine!" What could I say?

It was the most memorable holiday. Kids brightened up as I made my Santa rounds. Finally, the last child was gifted and my tour was over. A few months later, I married the play and recreation director, continuing with many more years of playing Santa to our 6 children. I will never forget that first accidental substitution that changed my life.

Roger J. Meyer, MD
Poulsbo, WA

Endless stories come to mind from my days on the Navajo Indian reservation. One afternoon the ambulance brought in a very dehydrated baby from the field. I was told that they had responded to smoke signals. "C'mon, you've got to be kidding. It's the 1980s!" It turns out that the baby's grandmother was caring for him alone in her very isolated hogan. She knew he was getting in trouble from his diarrhea and lack of intake. Unfortunately, one of the rather infrequent rainstorms had turned the road to her hogan into a mass of impassable mud. She built a big fire and used a blanket to make a "signal" of distress. Sure enough, at the trading post 10 or 20 miles away it was spotted. No matter how isolated, the Navajo always knew about their neighbors.

Peter D. Grundl, MD
Falls Church, VA

I recall years ago when a young mother and her 4-year-old daughter, Lisa, came into the office for a minor illness. In the course of the visit the mother remarked that the little girl's daddy was in the hospital because of a car accident. I asked, "How badly was he hurt?" The mother replied, "Well, fortunately his head wasn't hurt, but he fractured his legs, some ribs, and his left wrist." I replied, "That's terrible." And before I could say more, little Lisa said in a very authoritative voice, "But Dr 'Ebers,' he is still good looking."

Joseph C. Evers, MD
McLean, VA

Four-year-old Josh visited his 89-year-old great-grand-mother, who is bedridden, very frail, and does not talk anymore. After looking at her and gently touching and stroking her hand he commented, "It is sad to get old."

Claus Helbing, MD
Annandale, VA

✆

I will never forget 3-year-old Ben who, when I had just come on service as a pediatric fellow in hematology, needed outpatient intrathecal (injection through lumbar puncture) treatment for the leukemic cells in his cerebrospinal fluid after his disease had otherwise gone into remission.

When I informed his mother that the nurse had said it would be 20 minutes before she could help me with the lumbar puncture, his mother said, "You don't need a nurse. Ben has had this before," and turning to Ben, "You'll be fine won't you?" He nodded somberly and walked toward the treatment room.

There were just the 2 of us in the room. After I had helped him take off his tartan pants and weskit, his crisp white shirt, and little tartan bow tie, he dutifully climbed up on the examining table and lay down in a fetal position, his back to me. He whimpered a bit with the local anesthetic and a bit more when I injected the drug that must have burned terribly, but he never moved.

When it was finished, and I had helped him down off the table and into his little plaid outfit, he stuck out his hand to shake hands and said, "Thank you very much."

It was suddenly difficult to find the way back to his mother because I was struggling so hard to hold back the tears. The next 20 minutes were spent alone in the treatment room weeping because I knew that in those days (1960s), surviving acute lymphocytic leukemia was very rare.

I never saw Ben again and do not know what his outcome was. I have often wondered, though, if I were to develop a terminal illness whether I could deal with it like Ben. I do know that I would be thinking about his courage all the way through. He gave me a wonderful gift.

Beverley J. Bayes, MD
McLean, VA

℘

There was a little boy, age 6, who had been placed in the pediatric intensive care unit for observation after a head injury in which he had lost consciousness. When I came on duty at 8:00 am and made my rounds, I asked him if he had slept well. He very sternly said, "I would have slept better if they hadn't played those video games all night long."

He was, of course, referring to the monitors and dinamap machines. I had to share this with my colleagues because we often think of the sights and sounds around us as "normal."

Mary Williamson, RN
Falls Church, VA

Teachings From Children and About Them

From Children

- Never trust a dog to watch your food.
- When your dad is really mad and asks you, "Do I look stupid?" don't give an honest answer.
- Never ask for anything that costs more than 5 dollars when your parents are doing the taxes.
- When you get a bad grade in school, show it to your mom when she's on the phone.
- If you really want a kitten, start out by asking for a horse.
- You can never hide a piece of broccoli in a glass of milk.
- When your mom is mad at your dad, don't let her brush your hair.
- Don't pull your granddad's finger when he asks you to.
- Never, ever tell your mom her diet isn't working.

About Children

- Having a child fall asleep in your arms is one of the most peaceful experiences in the world.
- Never say no to a gift from a child.
- Childhood is like a roll of toilet paper...the closer it gets to the end, the faster it goes.
- You know you are hooked for life when your newborn granddaughter holds your little finger for the first time.
- In any dispute with your child, it is better to be kind than to be right.

Gathered by
James A. Stockman III, MD
Chapel Hill, NC

Submissions

If you have a personal anecdote that you would like to submit for a future edition of *The Joys of Pediatrics,* please send it via e-mail to joysofpeds@aap.org or by mail to

American Academy of Pediatrics
Attn: Publications Dept
141 Northwest Point Blvd
Elk Grove Village, IL 60007-1098

American Academy of Pediatrics

The American Academy of Pediatrics (AAP) and its member pediatricians dedicate their efforts and resources to the health, safety, and well-being of infants, children, adolescents, and young adults. The AAP has approximately 60,000 members in the United States, Canada, and Latin America. Members include pediatricians, pediatric medical subspecialists, and pediatric surgical specialists. More than 34,000 members are board certified and called Fellows of the AAP (FAAP).

Core Values. We believe:
- In the inherent worth of all children; they are our most enduring and vulnerable legacy.
- Children deserve optimal health and the highest quality health care.
- Pediatricians are the best qualified to provide child health care.

The American Academy of Pediatrics is the organization to advance child health and well-being.

Vision. Children have optimal health and well-being and are valued by society. Academy members practice the highest quality health care and experience professional satisfaction and personal well-being.

Mission. The mission of the American Academy of Pediatrics is to attain optimal physical, mental, and social health and well-being for all infants, children, adolescents, and young adults. To accomplish this mission, the Academy shall support the professional needs of its members.